The Complete Guide to Echocardiography

David I. Silverman, MD
Professor of Medicine
University of Connecticut School of Medicine
Director, Echocardiography Laboratory
Hartford Hospital
Hartford, CT

Warren J. Manning, MD
Professor of Medicine and Radiology
Harvard Medical School
Section Chief, Non-invasive Cardiac Imaging
Beth Israel Deaconess Medical Center
Boston, MA

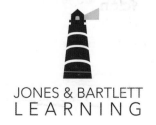

JONES & BARTLETT
L E A R N I N G

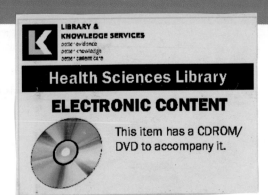

World Headquarters

Jones & Bartlett Learning
40 Tall Pine Drive
Sudbury, MA 01776
978-443-5000
info@jblearning.com
www.jblearning.com

Jones & Bartlett Learning
Canada
6339 Ormindale Way
Mississauga, Ontario L5V 1J2
Canada

Jones & Bartlett Learning
International
Barb House, Barb Mews
London W6 7PA
United Kingdom

Jones & Bartlett Learning books and products are available through most bookstores and online booksellers. To contact Jones & Bartlett Learning directly, call 800-832-0034, fax 978-443-8000, or visit our website, www.jblearning.com.

Substantial discounts on bulk quantities of Jones & Bartlett Learning publications are available to corporations, professional associations, and other qualified organizations. For details and specific discount information, contact the special sales department at Jones & Bartlett Learning via the above contact information or send an email to specialsales@jblearning.com.

The authors, editor, and publisher have made every effort to provide accurate information. However, they are not responsible for errors, omissions, or for any outcomes related to the use of the contents of this book and take no responsibility for the use of the products and procedures described. Treatments and side effects described in this book may not be applicable to all people; likewise, some people may require a dose or experience a side effect that is not described herein. Drugs and medical devices are discussed that may have limited availability controlled by the Food and Drug Administration (FDA) for use only in a research study or clinical trial. Research, clinical practice, and government regulations often change the accepted standard in this field. When consideration is being given to use of any drug in the clinical setting, the healthcare provider or reader is responsible for determining FDA status of the drug, reading the package insert, and reviewing prescribing information for the most up-to-date recommendations on dose, precautions, and contraindications, and determining the appropriate usage for the product. This is especially important in the case of drugs that are new or seldom used.

Production Credits
Executive Publisher: Christopher Davis
Editorial Assistant: Sara Cameron
Associate Production Editor: Jill Morton
Marketing Manager: Rebecca Rockel
V.P., Manufacturing and Inventory Control: Therese Connell
Composition: Shawn Girsberger
Cover Design: Scott Moden
Cover Image: Courtesy of Warren Manning, MD
Assistant Photo Researcher: Rebecca Ritter
Printing and Binding: Replika Press Pvt. Ltd.
Cover Printing: Replika Press Pvt. Ltd.

Library of Congress Cataloging-in-Publication Data
Silverman, David I.
  The complete guide to echocardiography / by David I. Silverman and Warren J. Manning.
     p. ; cm.
  Includes bibliographical references and index.
  ISBN-13: 978-0-7637-8405-8
  ISBN-10: 0-7637-8405-2
  1. Echocardiography—Examinations, questions, etc. I. Manning, Warren J. II. Title.
  [DNLM: 1. Echocardiography—Examination Questions. WG 18.2]
  RC683.5.U5S55 2012
  616.1′207543076—dc22
                            2010036582

6048
Printed in India
14 13 12 11 10   10 9 8 7 6 5 4 3 2 1

For Gabriel and Alexandra

For Sue, Anya, Sara, Isaac, and Elie

CONTENTS

PREFACE

This book is intended to help readers gain mastery of the essential visual elements of echocardiography in combination with an understanding of anatomy, hemodynamics, pathophysiology, and disease recognition. Each chapter begins with a few questions to help you focus on the topic. The chapters are presented in a series of numbered sections to allow for easy reference. Essential concepts are placed in *italics*. At the end of each chapter, board review–style questions are presented, followed by detailed answers with reference to the specific section within the chapter that covers the topic. In addition to the written and visual material presented in the text, the accompanying CD-ROM provides a video clip library of two-dimensional, M-mode, and Doppler images organized in parallel to each chapter. These features, referred to as Learning Directives, are denoted throughout the text by this icon: .

Although this book provides a broad overview of topics in echocardiography, despite its title, it is not meant to be exhaustive. Given that one of its core missions is to provide an efficient and focused tool for review and preparation for the ASCexam and ReASCexam, it concentrates on topics covered by the exam and described on the National Board of Echocardiography's Web site (www.echoboards.org/ascexam/out-line.html). The questions are intentionally designed to be challenging and to test your knowledge at the advanced level that will be required to pass the exam.

A few editorial notes about the business of learning to interpret an echocardiographic study: While the didactic/scholarly portion of echocardiography has markedly increased since its inception, it remains our belief that echocardiography is fundamentally about reconstructing a three-dimensional structure (the heart) from two-dimensional images. As with all imaging techniques, pattern recognition is important. Whether an individual is cognitively gifted in this area or not, there is no substitute for viewing lots of images.

As with any accumulated skill, echocardiography is practice dependent. The more images you view, the more you can "see." Start by learning the breadth of *normal*, whether it is echocardiographic dimensions, anatomic placements, valvular gradients, or the many quantitative formulae. While you should not memorize every formula you see, a few calculations are critical to have at your mental fingertips, especially those for quantification of valvular stenosis and regurgitation. You want to incorporate the basic concepts of cardiac anatomy, physiology, and pathophysiology as part of your echocardiography skill set. That, by the way, will make you a better cardiologist overall!

For a thorough discussion and encyclopedia of normal values, the American Society of Echocardiography (ASE) article on quantitation on this subject is essential reading (Lang RE, Bierig M, Devereux RB, et al. Recommendations for chamber quantification: a report from the American Society of Echocardiography's Guidelines and Standards Committee and the Chamber Quantification Writing Group, developed in conjunction with the European Association of Echocardiography, a branch of the European Society of Cardiology. *J Am Soc Echocardiogr* 2005:18:1441–1463). Print it. Read it. Put it under your pillow. Then read it again. It is a treasure trove of essential echocardiography lore that you will employ on a daily basis.

The ASE Web site (www.asecho.org) is another terrific resource with a variety of primary and Continuing Medical Education teaching resources. It is also an organization worth joining.

Good luck. We hope we've made your trip along the path to echocardiography proficiency a little easier.

ACKNOWLEDGMENTS

The authors wish to thank Lee Goldman; Kyle Richards, MD; Eli Gelfand, MD; and the sonographers and cardiology fellows of Hartford Hospital and the Beth Israel Deaconess Medical Center for their invaluable technical and editorial assistance. We also thank our administrative assistants Clayre Johnson, at Hartford Hospital, and Iris Wasserman, at the Beth Israel Deaconess Medical Center, for their many efforts. Finally we thank Gabriel, Alexandra, Sue, Anya, Sara Yitz, and Elie for allowing us to undertake this additional task despite an already full schedule.

CONTRIBUTORS

David I. Silverman, MD
Professor of Medicine
University of Connecticut School of Medicine
Director, Echocardiography Laboratory
Hartford Hospital
Hartford, CT

Warren J. Manning, MD
Professor of Medicine and Radiology
Harvard Medical School
Section Chief, Non-invasive Cardiac Imaging
Beth Israel Deaconess Medical Center
Boston, MA

Chapter 12
Felice A. Heller, MD
Assistant Clinical Professor of Pediatrics
Director, Adult Congenital Heart Disease Program
Connecticut Children's Medical Center
Hartford, CT

ABBREVIATIONS

Ao	aorta
ASE	American Society of Echocardiography
dB	decibel
CW	continuous wave
EDD	end-diastolic dimension
EDP	end-diastolic pressure
ERO	effective regurgitant orifice
ESD	end-systolic dimension
Hz	hertz
ILWT	inferolateral wall thickness
IVC	inferior vena cava
IVCT	isovolumic contraction time
IVRT	isovolumic relaxation time
kHz	kilohertz
LA	left atrium
LV	left ventricle
LVOT	left ventricular outflow tract
MHz	megahertz
MV	mitral valve

PA	pulmonary artery
PFO	patent foramen ovale
PISA	proximal isovelocity surface area
PRF	pulse repetition frequency
PW	pulse wave
RA	right atrium
RV	right ventricle
RVOT	right ventricular outflow tract
SVC	superior vena cava
SWT	septal wall thickness
TDI	tissue Doppler imaging
TEE	transesophageal echocardiogram
TTE	transthoracic echocardiogram
2D	two dimensional
VTI	velocity time integral
$>$	greater than
$\geq$	greater than or equal to
$<$	less than
$\leq$	less than or equal to

1

PHYSICS, INSTRUMENTATION, AND CONTRAST

PRACTICE QUESTIONS

Q1.1 The four components of an ultrasound wave are:

a. Frequency, power, amplitude, wavelength

b. Propagation speed, power, amplitude, wavelength

c. Power, amplitude, propagation speed, frequency

d. Amplitude, wavelength, propagation speed, frequency

e. Wavelength, frequency, power, propagation speed

Q1.2 The frequency of an ultrasound beam is a function of the:

a. Transducer

b. Medium

c. Power supply

d. Pressure the sonographer applies to the chest

e. Transducer as well as the medium

Q1.3 Production of an ultrasound reflection depends upon a change in the:

a. Frequency of the waveform

b. Wavelength of the waveform

c. Propagation speed of the waveform

d. Pulse repetition frequency

e. Acoustic impedance of the medium

ANSWERS: 1.1. d; 1.2. a; 1.3. e

Properties of a Sound Wave

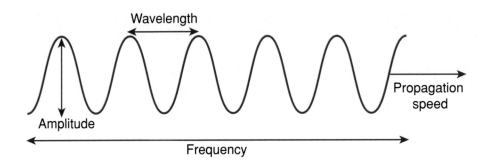

Figure 1.1   Properties of a sound wave.

1.1   The distance of one cycle from peak to peak is called the *wavelength* (Figure 1.1). The number of wavelengths that pass a given point per unit of time (e.g., per second) is the *frequency*. The velocity at which the waveform moves is the *propagation speed*. The height of the wave (from peak to trough) is the *amplitude*.

The trough, where pressure reaches a minimum, is called *rarefaction*, and the peak, where pressure reaches a maximum, is called *compression*. (These concepts become critical later when we talk about contrast).

1.2   Ultrasound differs from audible sound only in its frequency, and by definition begins at greater than 20,000 Hz, or greater than 20 kilohertz (kHz). Most transducer frequencies for human ultrasound imaging range from 1 to 10 megahertz (MHz).

Propagation speed is calculated as:

$$\text{propagation speed} = \text{wavelength} \times \text{frequency}$$

The frequency of an ultrasound wave is a function of the transducer and is fixed. It does not change. The unit for measuring frequency is cycles/sec, or hertz. The frequency of an ultrasound wave is usually measured in megahertz (MHz; mega $= 10^6$).

Period is the reciprocal of frequency, or 1/frequency.

Propagation speed is a function of the medium and is unique to any particular medium. As with frequency, it does not change (unless the wave passes from one medium to the next).

1.3 Two properties of the medium determine propagation speed: *density* (mass/volume) and *stiffness* (compressibility). *Their effects are opposite:*

- The *greater* the stiffness of the medium, the *faster* the propagation speed.

- The *greater* the density of the medium, the *slower* the propagation speed.

Thus, a biological material such as bone is a very fast conductor of sound because it is stiff but not dense. Air is a very slow conductor of sound because while it is not dense, it is not stiff either. In general, the progression of increasing propagation speed through biological media is:

air	lung	fat	muscle	bone

slowest   fastest

1.4 The ultrasound propagation speed in human tissue is 1540 m/sec (a number, alas, probably worth memorizing!). Wavelength is determined by both the transducer and the medium. Like propagation speed and frequency, it is fixed, with units in centimeters, millimeters, etc. From the previous equation:

$$\text{wavelength} = \text{propagation speed/frequency}$$

Therefore, if the frequency is 1 MHz, the wavelength is 1.54 mm; if the frequency is 2 MHz, the wavelength is 0.77 mm; etc.

Remember, none of these three variables change as the wave moves through tissue.

1.5 *Amplitude* is determined by the power applied to the piezoelectric crystal. Amplitude attenuates linearly with time/distance, and the *rate of attenuation is directly proportional to the frequency*. Units vary depending upon exactly what form the acoustic variable is being described in.

Variable	Unit
Distance	Centimeters, millimeters, etc.
Power	Watts/cm^2
Pressure	Pascal

1.6   *Attenuation* is the process by which amplitude, alone among the fundamental ultrasound variables, decreases with time. Attenuation is a function of several factors, including:

1.   The initial wave frequency. The higher the initial wave frequency, the *faster* the rate of attenuation.

2.   The initial wave amplitude. The higher the initial amplitude, the *slower* the rate of attenuation.

The attenuation coefficient describes the rate of attenuation/cm. Units are in decibels (dB), a unit measuring acoustic power or intensity that is represented along a relative logarithmic scale.

The rate of attenuation is also affected by the nature of the medium through which the sound wave is traveling. In general, the *greater* the density of the medium, the *slower* the rate of attenuation (with water < soft tissue << bone < air). This phenomenon explains in part why it is so difficult to produce a good echocardiogram in a patient with a barrel chest or hyperinflated lungs.

1.7   *Depth of penetration* is the distance at which intensity drops by half. Depth of penetration is inversely proportional to the attenuation coefficient.

Power is the amount of electrical energy applied to the system. Power can be expressed in several ways, but is usually defined in watts/cm^2. The most common (and useful) way to describe power is:

- power = intensity × beam area

- intensity = power/beam area

The unit for measuring power is watts/cm^2, and the normal range is 0.001–100 watts/cm^2.

Pressure: Sound waves are pressure waves. The unit of pressure commonly used is the pascal.

1.8   With the exception of continuous wave (CW) Doppler, all other forms of ultrasound are transmitted as discrete packets. Each packet has a *pulse length,* which is the actual length or distance the pulse occupies in space, usually measured in mm.

pulse length = number of cycles in a pulse × wavelength

The *pulse duration* is the time interval between the beginning of the generation of a pulse and the end of that pulse (or the time required to generate the pulse), measured in milliseconds. Pulse duration is inversely related to frequency; increasing frequency will shorten pulse duration.

1.9 *Pulse repetition frequency* (PRF) is the rate at which pulses are generated per unit of time. It is measured in cycles per second, or hertz (Hz). **Note that the PRF is different than the frequency of the wave, although they are interconnected, especially when it comes to Doppler.** Normal PRF is usually 1000–10,000 Hz, or 1–10 kHz.

Because the speed of ultrasound in tissue is fixed (1540 m/sec), knowing the distance a pulse has to travel to reach its target allows you to calculate the PRF as:

$$1 \text{ cycle} = \frac{2 \times \text{distance traveled in cm}}{154 \text{ cm/msec}} = \frac{\text{distance traveled}}{77 \text{cm/msec}}$$

or:

$$0.77/\text{distance in cm}$$

This formula gives you a PRF in kHz.

Unlike the frequency of the wave, the PRF will change under several conditions. Increasing the imaging depth will decrease the PRF because it will take longer for the signal to return to the transducer. Increasing the sample volume size will produce the same effect because now you are gathering more packets (and waiting for them to come back) before you send out the next group.

Pulse repetition period is the time from the start of one pulse to the next. This is the reciprocal of the PRF. Units are in seconds, milliseconds, etc. The pulse repetition period includes the time taken by the pulse (or pulse duration) and the "dead time" until the next pulse.

1.10 *Duty factor* is the time used to generate a pulse as a proportion of the total time. The duty factor is a percentage and can range from 100 (for CW Doppler) to 0 (no pulse generated).

Algebraically:

$$\text{duty factor} = \text{pulse duration/pulse repetition period}$$

or:

$$\text{pulse duration} \times \text{PRF}$$

1.11 *Spatial resolution* defines the distance between two points that can be resolved: the smaller the number, the better the spatial resolution. *Axial or longitudinal resolution* is related to both transducer frequency (and thus wavelength) and pulse length. In general, the axial resolution of most transthoracic echocardiogram (TTE) systems is about 2 mm.

$$\text{axial resolution} = \frac{\text{pulse length}}{2}$$
$$= \frac{\text{number of cycles in pulse} \times \text{wavelength}}{2}$$

Or, algebraically:

$$\frac{0.77 \times \text{number of cycles in pulse}}{\text{frequency}}$$

Higher frequencies mean a shorter period, a shorter pulse duration (usually), and a shorter spatial pulse length. They also mean a shorter penetration because attenuation is greater at higher frequencies.

Lateral resolution is related to beam width; the narrower the beam, the greater the resolution. Beam width is also a function of (1) frequency, (2) focal depth, (3) line density, and (4) lens size, so changing any of these parameters also changes lateral resolution.

Focusing

1.12 An ultrasound beam has all the characteristics of a beam of light. It produces a focal length inside of a focal zone with a near field and a far field (Figure 1.2). The focal length is a direct function of the square of the radius of curvature of the transducer and an inverse function of wavelength.

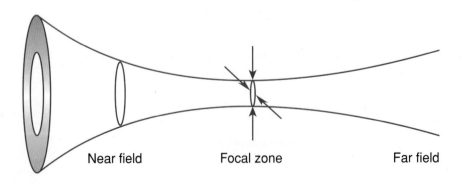

Near field   Focal zone   Far field

Figure 1.2   Characteristics of focusing.

The *focal length* is:

- Directly proportional to the radius of the transducer

- Directly proportional to the frequency

- Inversely proportional to the wavelength

Thus, increasing either the transducer diameter or transducer frequency will increase the focal length. Increasing the wavelength will decrease the focal length.

The size of the focal zone is:

- Directly proportional to the size the beam

- Directly proportional to the curvature of the lens (if one is used)

Focal length is calculated as:

$$\frac{\text{lens diameter}^2 \times \text{frequency}}{6}$$

Focusing can be accomplished by the following means (Figure 1.3):

1. Using an acoustic lens (analogous to optical focusing). This is usually referred to as fixed focusing and represents a fairly primitive technique that is seldom used currently.

2. Using an electronic "lens" by timing the firing of the elements in the transducer. This is referred to as mechanical focusing and is accomplished by using an annular-phased array transducer, the most common transducer type used currently.

3. Placing a curved mirror behind the crystal and firing toward it.

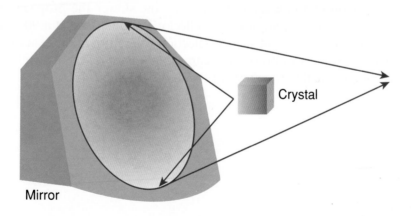

Figure 1.3 Focusing of an ultrasound beam using an acoustic mirror.

Steering the beam can be accomplished by varying the timing at which each signal within the array is either sent or received. Such variance is described as either transit time delay or receive time delay.

The Fate of Ultrasound

1.13   To paraphrase Woody Hayes' description of a forward pass, three things can happen, but only one of them is desirable (i.e., helps produce an image):

1.   *Absorption*: The wave disappears as it propagates as the result of attenuation.

2.   *Scattering*: The wave dissipates as it bounces off various minor reflectors. When the size of a single particle is quite small (ratio of circumference/wavelength < 1), a particular form of scattering called Rayleigh scattering occurs. Red blood cells fulfill this small size criterion and are therefore the prime source of Rayleigh scattering. Rayleigh scattering is the phenomenon in the electromagnetic world that explains why the sky is blue. Under some circumstances, especially when using contrast, scatter reflections can produce a useful image (more on this in the Contrast section).

3.   *Reflection*: The wave returns to the sound source. Reflection is preferred and occurs when there is a *change in the density of one medium to the next*, as from blood to muscle. These echoes are described as *specular*. Specular echoes are produced by surfaces of a sufficient size and smoothness. Note that specular reflection is also angle dependent; the wider the angle, the less effectively the reflected wave is returned to the transducer.

1.14   *Acoustic impedance* describes the resistance of a medium to the movement of sound through it. Its units are in rayls, and it is defined as density multiplied by propagation speed.

For a reflection to occur, there must be a change in the acoustic impedance of the medium. As discussed previously, the greater the density, the slower the propagation speed. Ideally, you want the ultrasound beam to reflect off an interface at a 90° angle since the laws of physics determine that such a reflection will return in the exact same direction from which it came. For ultrasound beams that do not reflect at a right angle, the angle of reflection is equal to the angle of incidence (Figure 1.4a).

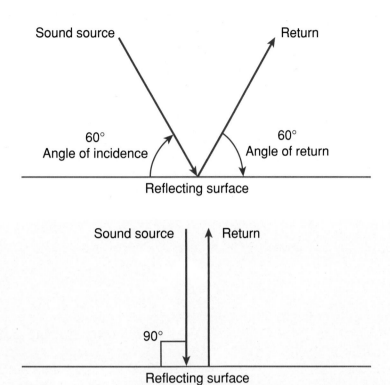

Figure 1.4a   Characteristics of the angle of reflection of an ultrasound beam. The angle of incident reflection determines the angle of return.

The *intensity reflection coefficient* is the percentage of ultrasound returned to the transducer and is calculated as:

$$\frac{\text{reflected intensity}}{\text{incident intensity}}$$

Or, where Z equals the impedance (in rayls):

$$\frac{(Z \text{ second layer} - Z \text{ 1st layer})^2}{(Z \text{ second layer} + Z \text{ 1st layer})^2}$$

Artifacts

1.15   Ultrasound imaging is associated with many artifacts that can be understood from basic physics.

Side lobes are created as unwanted "beamlets" on the edge of the central beam (Figure 1.4b). They are most common in transducers with a single small element or with linear-phased array transducers. They produce the optical effect of placing an image that is not real beside the real image or elongating the real image laterally.

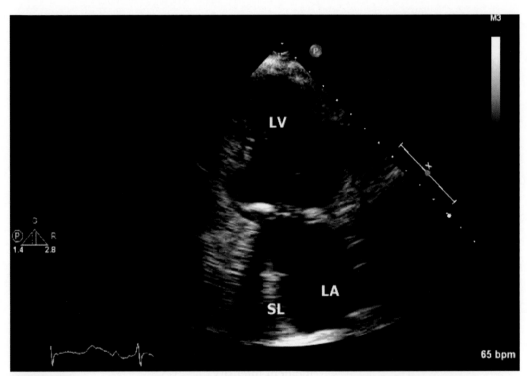

Figure 1.4b   A sidelobe (SL) artifact seen in the left atrium (LA). LV, left ventricle.

LEARNING DIRECTIVE

See Clip 1.7: A side-lobe artifact from the echodense noncoronary leaflet spreads into the echo-free space adjacent.

Reverberation or mirror artifacts occur as the result of a wave reflecting off a surface that it has already passed on its way back to the transducer. Because the sonograph uses total go-and-return time to calculate distance, the artifact will appear distal to the original surface at a distance that is equal to the interval between the original reflection and the reverberator (Figure 1.5).

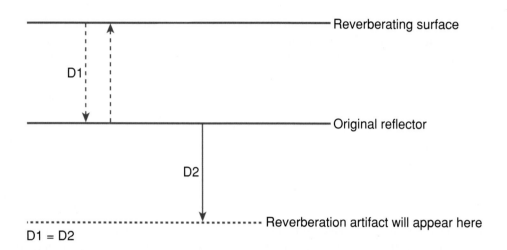

Figure 1.5   The geometry of a reverberation artifact. The time required for the ultrasound beam to reverberate between the two surfaces will place the artifact at a distance on the screen that is a mathematical multiple of that original distance.

LEARNING DIRECTIVE

See Clip 1.6: A mirror artifact in the posterior left atrium moves in the direction opposite its reflector, the anterior mitral leaflet.

Acoustic shadow artifact occurs when a proximal reflector excludes the transmission of echoes behind it. Any strong reflector, such as calcium and prosthetic heart valves, will produce this phenomenon.

Ghosting artifact occurs when the motion of a valve or other rapidly moving structure creates enough blood movement to produce a brief flash of color that does not represent true blood flow.

Transducers

1.16   Transducers are comprised of several parts.

1. *Piezoelectric crystal*: Vibrates at a characteristic frequency. Piezoelectric crystals can be made from a variety of materials. The thickness of the material determines the characteristic frequency. Thickness and frequency are inversely proportional.

2. *Matching layer*: Allows transmission from the transducer into the body through a layer whose impedance is midway between the two with a minimum loss of power. Its purpose is to minimize unwanted reflections from the patient. An ideal matching layer allows one-quarter of the wavelength initially produced by the transducer.

3. *Damping element, or backing layer*: Shortens the pulse duration and pulse length, improves longitudinal resolution, and prevents backward transmission of the wave.

4. *Case and power supply*

1.17 *Dynamic range* describes the spectrum of signals captured by the transducer upon their return. Because of attenuation, objects that are farther away produce ultrasound packets with smaller amplitude. To avoid trying to interpret miniscule signals of minimal amplitude, the detection device limits the range of signals it processes. Dynamic range is measured in decibels, which is a unit that describes the magnitude of the pressure wave that produces sound. Decibels (dB) are measured on a log scale as the ratio of one power (or intensity) to another, or to a reference unit. The range of most transducers is 100 dB (or 100,000 to 1). The dynamic range of most display systems is only 30 dB, so the received signals must undergo a process of *acoustic compression* in which the entire range is fit onto the scale of the receiving device and extraneous (low-intensity) signals are rejected.

1.18 What happens after a signal returns to the transducer?

1. *Amplification*: With attenuation, the signal that returns is weak and must be boosted. This can be accomplished by the sonographer. Units are in dB. This process is controlled by turning the gain up or down. In this process, *all echoes are boosted equally*.

LEARNING DIRECTIVE

See Clip 1.2: An image that is deliberately overgained. The increase in gain causes not only increased echodensity but also a spreading of the boundaries of the structure of the image.

2. *Compensation*: Distant signals are weaker and must be boosted through this process. This is what the time-gain-compensation (TGC) levers do. Today, lateral gain compensation (LGC) allows for the same process from side to side.

3. *Compression*: This setting of the dynamic range (see Section 1.17) is done in an automated fashion by the sonographer. Dynamic range is narrower for two-dimensional (2D) than M-mode.

4. *Demodulation*: The relevant information is extracted for the imaging device or scan converter.

5. *Rejection*: This process removes low-amplitude echoes (noise) below a certain threshold.

1.19   Once all postprocessing has occurred, the signal enters a scan converter that transforms the signal into a gray scale and stores it. Most current scan converters use digital processing, converting the information in each pixel into a binary number.

Next, the signal is transferred electronically to a display device, either analogue (cathode ray tube) or digital (LCD panel). Each pixel created by the scan converter is displayed. The display device usually allows for adjustment of brightness and contrast. Image resolution depends upon the same variables that affect any display, in particular the number of pixels in the picture and the number of scan lines transmitted and received.

1.20   So far we have talked about one packet of ultrasound at a time. In reality, the transducer sends out packets in series one after the other in scan lines. The picture you receive depends upon:

1. The number of scan lines sent per unit of time

2. The width of the scan or sector angle

3. The distance each scan line travels (imaging depth)

4. The PRF of each scan line

5. The frame rate or number of individual frames collected per unit of time to make the picture (just like in the movies)

All of these factors affect the *temporal resolution* of the scan. Characteristics of temporal resolution include:

1. Decreases with increasing scan lines (more information to gather)

2. Decreases with increasing sector width

3. Decreases with increasing imaging depth

4. Decreases with increasing sector size

Bioeffects

1.21   Ultrasound bioeffects come in two forms, thermal (which can produce *heating*) and mechanical (which can produce *cavitation*). The amount of acoustic energy applied depends upon two factors, the intensity of the beam being applied and the amount of time the pulse is on. These factors can be described by both their average and peak values in the following fashion:

1.   *Spatial average intensity* is defined as power/transducer surface area.

2.   *Spatial peak intensity* describes the portion of the beam (usually the center) that generates the greatest energy.

3.   *Temporal average intensity* is the average intensity received by the tissue.

4.   *Temporal peak intensity* is the peak intensity that tissue is exposed to during a pulse.

The total energy applied is estimated by combining both spatial and temporal factors. For example, spatial peak–temporal peak (SPTP) intensity is measured as the peak intensity during a pulse. By contrast, spatial average–temporal average (SATA) intensity is measured as the average intensity during a pulse. Because no energy is being applied when the pulse is off, temporal intensity is defined by the duty factor. CW Doppler produces higher temporal intensities than PW Doppler or ultrasound because the pulse is always on.

Contrast

1.22   Contrast comes in two basic forms. The first is just agitated saline, which serves as a short-lived but effective opacifier of the right heart. (The other form of contrast is discussed in Section 1.24.) Agitated saline is used commonly for the identification of right-to-left intracardiac shunts, such as a patent foramen ovale (PFO) or atrial septal defect. Depending upon the size of the defect and the pressure difference across the interatrial septum, venous bolus injection of 4–5 cc of agitated saline will result in the premature appearance (within three beats of right heart opacification) of bubbles in the left atrium (LA) and left ventricle (LV). The number of bubbles passing into the LA with each heartbeat roughly corresponds to the size of the PFO, with more than 10 bubbles suggesting the diameter is > 4 mm. Many patients will only pass bubbles with cough or with Valsalva, so these maneuvers should be attempted in all conscious patients. If the passage of bubbles is delayed by six beats or more, the shunt is likely to be intrapulmonary.

The most common indication for this type of injection is for investigating the cardiac source of embolism in cryptogenic stroke. The association between PFO and stroke has been studied extensively but has yet to provide a clear consensus with regard to causality or treatment. The weight of the data suggests causal relationship for PFO in younger patients with cryptogenic stroke, but the optimal therapy for these patients remains elusive.

1.23   The other important result that saline contrast can produce is a *negative contrast effect* in which the left-to-right flow of blood across an atrial septal defect produces a focal echolucent area on the right-atrial side of the septum, clearing contrast in the area of flow (Figure 1.6). The major obstacle to this technique, and a cause of false-positive studies that you must guard against, is competitive flow from the inferior vena cava. Saline contrast is used with both TTE and transesophageal echocardiograms (TEE).

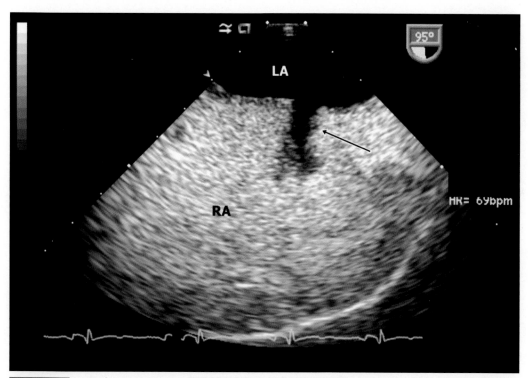

Figure 1.6   TEE in the midesophageal view demonstrates negative contract (arrow) in a patient with a secundum atrial septal defect and left-to-right flow. LA, left atrium; RA right atrium.

1.24   Microbubbles filled with an inert gas such as perflutren are the other form of contrast readily used in clinical echocardiography. Gas-filled microbubbles present a unique interface for ultrasound waves. Unlike most media, they are deformed by the wave itself, and they generate a secondary signal that can be interpreted by the transducer upon its return (Figure 1.7).

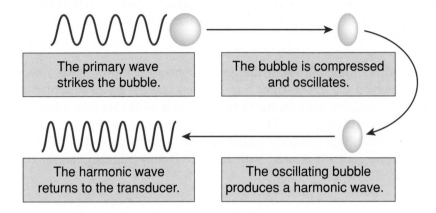

Figure 1.7   The physics of gas-filled microbubble contrast.

Harmonic waves are caused by a change in the shape of the wave's rarefaction and compression as it bounces off of the oscillating bubble. In so doing, the frequency of the wave changes slightly as a mathematical multiple of the original wave as it bounces off, and the phase (negative amplitude as compared to positive amplitude) may shift as well (Figure 1.8).

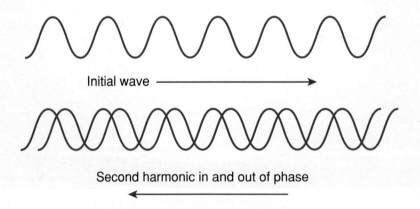

Figure 1.8   Harmonic waves in and out of phase.

The transducer can filter out the initial wave and listen only for the harmonic, and can add or subtract the waves in and out of phase to produce a coherent image. The other useful characteristic of reflective waves generated by harmonics is that they tend to be *nonlinear*. *Pulse inversion* is the technique for enhancing harmonics in which waves of alternating phases are transmitted. Because the frequency of fundamental waves is unchanged, the returning fundamental waves will tend to cancel each other out, while the nonlinear harmonic waves will be detected.

1.25   Harmonic imaging, which is used in most noncontrast clinical imaging, has multiple advantages over fundamental imaging. Fundamental imaging depends upon reflection off of *specular reflectors*, in which the wavelength is smaller than the size of the reflecting surface. These reflectors will produce strong echoes of the same frequency but only when the reflecting surface is perpendicular to the beam. Thus, fundamental imaging is a relatively poor technique for imaging parallel structures such as the lateral wall of the LV and septum in the apical four-chamber view, and it produces substantial artifact, especially in the near field of view. Because the surface area of *scatter reflectors* is smaller than the wavelength, the resulting angle of reflection is variable and the signal strength is weak. Nevertheless, specular reflectors will produce better echoes off of nonperpendicular surfaces and eliminate the *near-field clutter* seen commonly with fundamental imaging.

1.26   Contrast images using harmonics are best produced under the following conditions:

1. The proper acoustic pressure is used. Use too little acoustic pressure, and the bubbles will not resonate. Use too much acoustic pressure, and the bubbles will burst. Acoustic pressure is described by the *mechanical index*, which is defined as *acoustic power divided by the square root of frequency*. The mechanical index is controlled by the sonographer. When acoustic pressure is too high, the image will produce an artifact known as *swirling* (Figure 1.9).

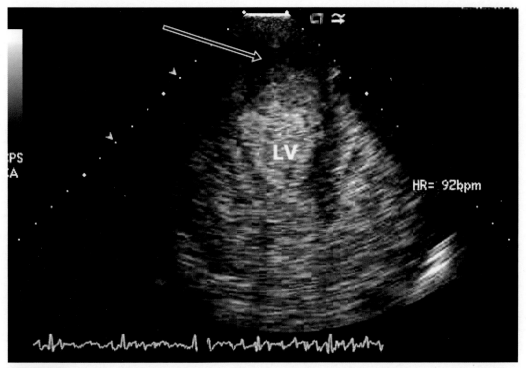

Figure 1.9   TTE in the apical four-chamber view demonstrates swirling artifact from a mechanical index set too high. Note the clear space at the apex (arrow).

LEARNING DIRECTIVE

See Clip 1.1: Swirling artifact during contrast injection caused by a mechanical index that is set too high.

2. The proper dose or infusion rate is used. Excessive infusion rates tend to produce the other major contrast artifact, *attenuation*. With attenuation, the distal area being imaged tends to produce dropout. To reduce attenuation, either turn down the infusion rate or reduce the volume of the bolus.

3. The midfield is imaged. Midfield images are best produced by harmonics because that is the distance at which the nonlinear response is produced.

4. Lower transmit frequencies are used.

1.27   Common uses of echocardiographic contrast include:

1. Two adjacent nonvisualized LV segments

2. Poorly visualized cardiac mass

3. Assessment of apical LV thrombus

4. LV pseudoaneurysm

5. Enhancement of spectral Doppler

1.28   Perflutren,[1] the commonly used contrast agent, is very safe but is contraindicated in certain subsets of patients, particularly those with large right-to-left or bidirectional intracardiac shunts. Perflutren should be used with caution in patients with pulmonary hypertension or in the setting of acute myocardial infarction or coronary instability. Under such circumstances, vital signs, oxygen saturation levels, and cardiac rhythm should be monitored for 30 minutes following injection. Allergic reactions should be treated as appropriate depending upon their level of severity.

---

1. (Definity, Lanthus Medical Imaging, Billerica, MA)

ADVANCED QUESTIONS

Q1.4   Which postprocessing technique produces an image with uniform brightness?

   a.   Amplification

   b.   Rejection

   c.   Compression

   d.   Compensation

   e.   Demodulation

Q1.5   Axial resolution is a function of:

   a.   Frequency

   b.   Amplitude

   c.   Propagation speed

   d.   Duty factor

   e.   Beam width

Q1.6   If the wavelength of an ultrasound beam is 2 mm, the frequency of the beam is:

   a.   0.38 MHz

   b.   0.77 MHz

   c.   1.54 MHz

   d.   2.31 MHz

   e.   Undefined from the information provided

Q1.7   Lateral resolution is a function of:

a.   Frequency

b.   Amplitude

c.   Propagation speed

d.   Duty factor

e.   Beam width

Q1.8   Which conditions will provide the best temporal resolution of an image?

a.   Wide sector width, shallow imaging depth

b.   Narrow sector width, deep imaging depth

c.   Wide sector width, deep imaging depth

d.   Narrow sector width, shallow imaging depth

Q1.9   The focal length of an ultrasound beam is a function of:

a.   Lens diameter and imaging depth

b.   Lens diameter and frequency

c.   Lens diameter and amplitude

d.   Amplitude and frequency

e.   Depth of penetration and duty factor

Q1.10   The function of the damping element within an ultrasound transducer is to:

a.   Absorb undesirable reflected wavelengths

b.   Prevent overheating

c.   Define the dynamic range of reflected wavelengths

d.   Limit unwanted reflection of wavelengths returning to the transducer

e.   Selectively amplify low-amplitude signals returning to the transducer

Q1.11   The focal length of an ultrasound transducer is:

    a.   Directly proportional to its radius of curvature and directly proportional to its frequency

    b.   Directly proportional to its radius of curvature and inversely proportional to its frequency

    c.   Inversely proportional to its radius of curvature and inversely proportional to its frequency

    d.   Inversely proportional to its radius of curvature and directly proportional to its frequency

Q1.12   Acoustic signals attenuate as they pass through a medium so that the amplitude of a wave reflecting off an object in the far field is smaller than a wave reflecting off an object in the near field. The postprocessing operation that differentially increases the amplitude of these weaker signals is referred to as:

    a.   Amplification

    b.   Compensation

    c.   Demodulation

    d.   Rejection

    e.   Compression

Q1.13   The distance from a reverberation artifact and the real structure that generates it is:

    a.   One-quarter the distance from the transducer to the real structure

    b.   One-half the distance from the transducer to the real structure

    c.   The distance from the transducer to the real structure

    d.   Four times the distance from the transducer to the real structure

    e.   Eight times the distance from transducer to the real structure

Q1.14 The density of the medium through which an ultrasound beam is traveling affects both its propagation speed and its rate of attenuation. The statement that best describes the relationship between the density of an ultrasound medium, the propagation speed, and the rate of attenuation of an ultrasound wave passing through it is:

a. The greater the medium density, the faster the propagation speed but the slower the rate of attenuation.

b. The greater the medium density, the faster the propagation speed and the faster the rate of attenuation.

c. The greater the medium density, the slower the propagation speed but the faster the rate of attenuation.

d. The greater the medium density, the slower the propagation speed and the slower the rate of attenuation.

Q1.15 The relationship between transducer frequency, longitudinal (axial) resolution, and depth of penetration can be best described as:

a. As transducer frequency increases, depth of penetration and axial resolution increase.

b. As transducer frequency increases, depth of penetration increases and axial resolution decreases.

c. As transducer frequency increases, depth of penetration decreases and axial resolution increases.

d. As transducer frequency increases, depth of penetration and axial resolution decrease.

e. As transducer frequency increases, depth of penetration and axial resolution remain unchanged.

Q1.16 Propagation speed increases with:

a. Increased density and decreased stiffness

b. Increased density and increased stiffness

c. Decreased density and increased stiffness

d. Decreased density and decreased stiffness

Q1.17 Wavelength is a function of the:

    a. Transducer

    b. Medium

    c. Transducer and the medium

    d. Neither the transducer nor the medium

Q1.18 The duty factor of a CW Doppler signal is:

    a. 25%

    b. 50%

    c. 75%

    d. 100%

    e. Not enough information is provided to answer this question.

Q1.19 Which component of an ultrasound transducer is designed to ensure that an adequate pulse is transmitted from the transducer to the skin?

    a. Piezoelectric crystal

    b. Case

    c. Wire

    d. Matching layer

    e. Damping material

Q1.20 The rate of attenuation of an ultrasound wave:

    a. Is directly related to its frequency and inversely related to its initial amplitude

    b. Is inversely related to its frequency and directly related to its initial amplitude

    c. Is directly related to both its frequency and its amplitude

    d. Is inversely related to both its frequency and its amplitude

    e. Has no relation to either frequency or amplitude

Q1.21   Which reflectors are most useful when produced by harmonic imaging?

    a.   Specular reflectors

    b.   Scatter reflectors

    c.   Pulse inversion reflectors

    d.   Autocorrelation reflectors

    e.   Primary frequency reflectors

Q1.22   TTE demonstrates a potential cardiac source of embolism in what percentage of stroke patients:

    a. $< 2\%$

    b.   7%

    c.   15%

    d.   25%

    e.   50%

Q1.23   Diagnostic criteria for atrial septal aneurysm, as depicted in the diagram in Figure Q1.23, consist of?

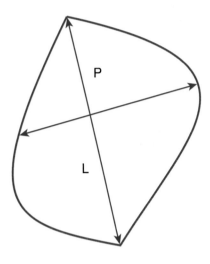

Figure Q1.23

a. $L \geq 5$ mm; $P \geq 10$ mm

b. $L \geq 10$ mm; $P \geq 10$ mm

c. $L \geq 10$ mm; $P \geq 5$ mm

d. $L \geq 10$ mm; $P \geq 20$ mm

e. $L \geq 20$ mm; $P \geq 20$ mm

Q1.24   Harmonic imaging:

a.   Increases near-field clutter

b.   Increases endocardial surface thickness

c.   Requires a narrow bandwidth

d.   Can only be used in conjunction with a contrast agent

e.   Filters for specular reflectors

Q1.25   Which of the following artifacts are produced during injection of echocardiographic contrast material?

a. Heating and cavitation

b. Mirror and reduplication

c. Side-lobe and acoustic shadow

d. Refraction and backscatter

e. Attenuation and swirling

ANSWERS

Q1.4   d: Compensation can produce uniform brightness by differentially increasing the gain of a selected area. Amplification uniformly increases the gain of the entire image. The other postprocessing techniques mentioned have no effect upon brightness. (Section **1.18**)

Q1.5   a: Axial resolution is a function of frequency or any surrogate in which frequency is contained such as pulse duration. Choice e, beam width, is the determining factor for lateral resolution. The other answers do not affect resolution of any type. (Section **1.11**)

Q1.6   b

$$\text{frequency} = \frac{\text{propagation speed}}{\text{wavelength}}$$
$$= \frac{1540 \text{ m/sec}}{0.002 \text{ m/cycle}}$$
$$= 7700 \text{ cycles/sec}$$
$$= 0.77 \text{ MHz}$$

(Section **1.4**)

Q1.7   e: See Question **1.5** and Section **1.11**.

Q1.8   d: The less information you gather and the faster you gather it, the higher the temporal resolution. (Section **1.20**)

Q1.9   b: This is a straightforward equation:

$$\text{focal length} = \frac{\text{lens diameter}^2 \times \text{frequency}}{6}$$

(Section **1.12**)

Q1.10   d: The damping layer shortens the pulse duration and prevents unwanted reflection of the returning signal by closely matching the density of the transducer. (Section **1.16**)

Q1.11   a: See Question **1.6** and Section **1.13**.

Q1.12   b: The key word here is differentially. Amplification uniformly increases signal amplitude. (Section **1.11**)

Q1.13   c: Reverberation artifact occurs when a pulse reflects off two reflectors before returning to the transducer. The back-and-forth trip doubles the time and therefore doubles the distance. (Section **1.15**)

Q1.14   d: Ultrasound waves move slowly through dense media but they also attenuate slowly. (Sections **1.3** and **1.5**)

Q1.15   c: High-frequency transducers provide excellent resolution but shallow imaging depth because the wave attenuates relatively rapidly. (Sections **1.6** and **1.11**)

Q1.16   c: Propagation speed is inversely proportional to density and directly proportional to stiffness. (Section **1.3**)

Q1.17   c: Because wavelength is related to both propagation speed and frequency, it depends upon both medium and transducer. (Sections **1.2** and **1.4**)

Q1.18   d: Duty factor describes the percentage of time between pulses during which a pulse is transmitted. Because CW Doppler transmits continuously, the percentage is 100. (Section **1.10**)

Q1.19   d: The matching layer prevents reflection by matching the impedance of the piezoelectric crystal. (Section **1.16**)

Q1.20   a: The higher the initial frequency, the faster the rate of attenuation. The higher the initial amplitude, the slower the rate of attenuation. (Section **1.6**)

Q1.21   b: See Section **1.25**.

Q1.22   b: TTE is a poor test for identification of cardiac source of embolism, despite the frequency with which it is ordered. (Section **1.22**)

Q1.23   b: Commonly accepted criteria for atrial septal aneurysm are a length ≥ 10 mm and a maximal bowing ≥ 10 mm. (Section **1.22**)

Q1.24   b: Harmonic imaging increases endocardial thickness because it returns scattered reflections. It reduces near-field clutter and requires a wide bandwidth. (Sections **1.24** and **1.25**)

Q1.25   e: See Section **1.26**.

2

THE NORMAL TWO-DIMENSIONAL ECHOCARDIOGRAPHIC EXAMINATION

Q2.1 In which view is the posterior leaflet of the tricuspid valve visualized?

a. Subcostal long axis

b. Parasternal short axis

c. Right ventricular inflow

d. Apical four-chamber

e. Apical five-chamber

Q2.2 From the parasternal long axis view, a pericardial effusion can reliably be distinguished from a pleural effusion by the:

a. Location of the inferior vena cava (IVC) in relation to the effusion

b. Location of the superior vena cava (SVC) in relation to the effusion

c. Location of the ascending aorta in relation to the effusion

d. Location of the descending aorta in relation to the effusion

e. Presence of thrombus within the effusion

Q2.3   To correct the parasternal long axis shown in Figure Q2.3:

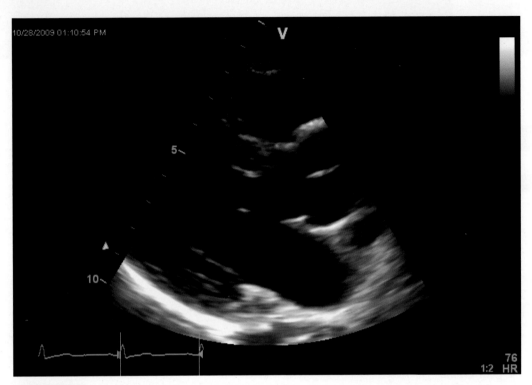

Figure Q2.3

a. Move the transducer up one intercostal space.

b. Move the transducer down one intercostal space.

c. Tilt the head of the transducer upward and to the left.

d. Tilt the head of the transducer downward and to the right.

e. No correction is necessary. The view is accurately obtained from the appropriate position.

2.1   The normal 2D TTE exam consists of four basic views: parasternal, apical, subcostal, and suprasternal.

Parasternal: From the left of the sternum at the third or fourth intercostal space (Figures 2.1 and 2.2). Normal 2D measurements commonly come from this view but may also be made in the parasternal short axis view.

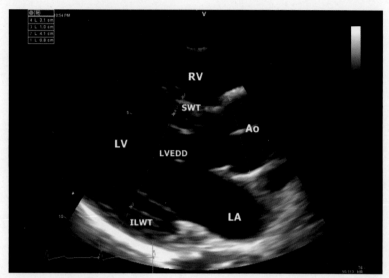

Figure 2.1   Normal TTE parasternal long axis view. The image is taken at the onset of the QRS complex (which does not necessarily produce the greatest LV diameter). The LV end-diastolic dimension (LVEDD), septal wall thickness (SWT), and inferolateral (formerly posterior) wall thickness (ILWT) are taken at a level just above the tips of the papillary muscles. Aortic root (Ao) dimensions at the sinus level are also taken during this phase of the cardiac cycle. Note that the mitral valve is open and aortic valve is closed.

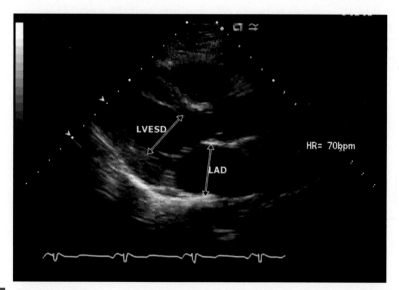

Figure 2.2   Normal TTE parasternal long axis end-systolic dimensions. The mitral valve is closed and the aortic valve is open. LVESD, left ventricular end-systolic dimension; LAD, left atrial dimension.

Normal 2D measurements are obtained in the parasternal long axis view from the third or fourth intercostal space. If the parasternal short axis view is used, make sure the measurements are still taken in parallel. Placing the transducer lower on the chest tilts the LV apex higher or more vertical on the screen (Figure 2.3).

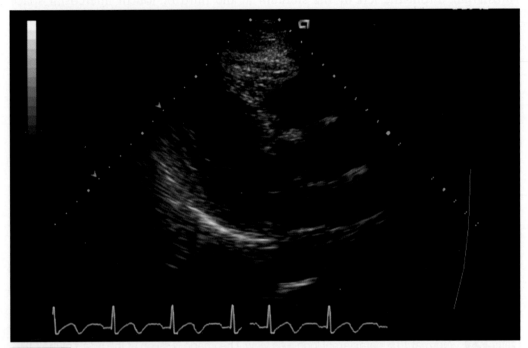

Figure 2.3   TTE parasternal long axis view. When the apex is tilted toward the top of the screen, the transducer has been placed an interspace or more too low.

2.2   A word on the "leading edge to leading edge" technique. The leading edge of an echo-reflector is the first surface the beam reflects off, and it produces the most faithful signal of the change between one medium and the next. This means the leading edge of any structure includes the wall of the structure on one side but not the other, because the first leading edge of the structure is measured on the outside and the second leading edge is measured on the inside, as shown in Figure 2.4.

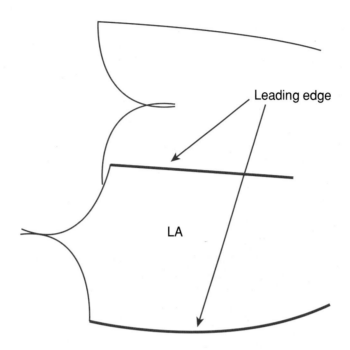

Figure 2.4   Schematic of the parasternal long axis view. The leading edge of the LA includes the wall of the aortic root.

For classic M-mode measurements of the LA and ascending aorta, the leading edge technique is used. Because both structures are thin walled, including the width of the proximal wall to the transducer does not alter the accuracy of the measurement. For internal dimensions, the thickness of the septum and inferolateral wall matter a great deal, so we use the trailing edge of the septum and the leading edge of the inferolateral wall. Nevertheless, when individuals use this nomenclature, they are referring to the dimensions as described initially.

2.3a   The *ascending aorta* is measured at the onset of the QRS complex, whereas the LA is measured at end-systole (maximal). The ascending aorta dimension is also measured in the parasternal long axis view. Measurements may be made at the level of the sinus of Valsalva, at the sinotubular junction, and at a level several centimeters above the sinotubular junction. For all measurements, data can be reported in absolute values or normalized for body surface area or height.

Wall thickness, LV volume, and LV mass are commonly normalized for body surface area, but can also be normalized weight or height alone.

Typical 2D measurements in a clinical exam include:

- Left ventricular end-diastolic dimension (LVEDD)

- Left ventricular end-systolic dimension (LVESD)

- Septal wall thickness (SWT)

- Inferolateral wall thickness (ILWT)

- Left atrial dimension (LAD)

- Aortic root diameter at the sinus level

LVEDD, SWT, ILWT, and aortic root are obtained at end-diastole (at QRS onset), whereas LVESD and the LAD are obtained at end-systole.

Normal 2D measurements for adults, as extracted from the American Society of Echocardiography (ASE) recommendations for chamber quantification, are (not accounting for body surface area) as follows:

	Men	Women
LAD	3.0–4.0 cm	2.7–3.8 cm
LVEDD	4.2–5.9 cm	3.9–5.3 cm
ILWT	0.6–1.0 cm	0.6–0.9 cm
SWT	0.6–1.0 cm	0.6–0.9 cm

2.3b The *descending aorta* is seen in cross section just below the LA and serves as a boundary between the pericardial and pleural spaces. Fluid collections between the LA and the descending aorta are pericardial, whereas fluid collections "behind" the aorta are pleural (Figure 2.5).

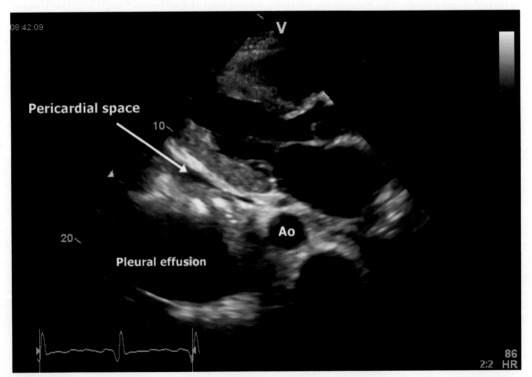

Figure 2.5 TTE parasternal long axis. The descending aorta (Ao) provides a boundary between the pleural effusion below and the pericardial space above.

2.4   From the parasternal long axis position, tilting the head of the transducer upward (toward the patient's head) and slightly to the left produces the *right ventricular inflow (RV) view*. This view can be used with Doppler to estimate the severity and peak flow velocity of tricuspid regurgitation, and, most critically, it is the only view in which the posterior tricuspid leaflet is well seen (Figure 2.6).

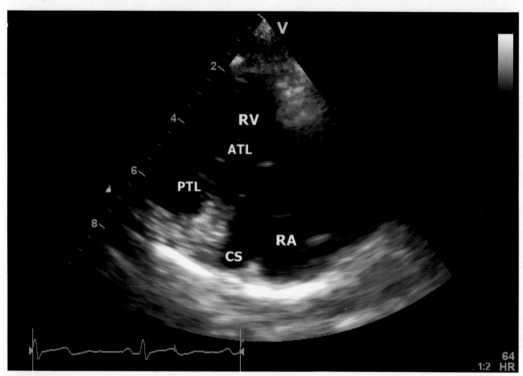

Figure 2.6   TTE in the right ventricular (RV) inflow view. The posterior tricuspid leaflet (PTL) is seen. The coronary sinus (CS) enters posteriorly. ATL, anterior tricuspid leaflet; RA, right atrium.

If the interventricular septum is in this view, you are off axis and the leaflet you are actually looking at is the septal leaflet (Figure 2.7).

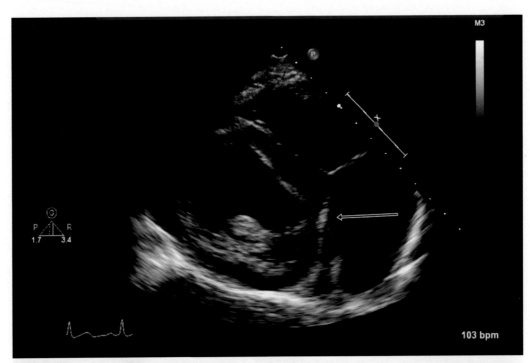

Figure 2.7   If the RV inflow view shows the interventricular septum, the septal leaflet of the tricuspid valve is visualized (arrow).

2.5   The parasternal short axis view at the level of the aortic valve depicts the anterior and septal tricuspid valve leaflets, all three aortic valve leaflets, two of three pulmonic valve leaflets, the right ventricle (RV) and right ventricular outflow tract (RVOT), and the right atrium (RA) and LA (Figure 2.8a).

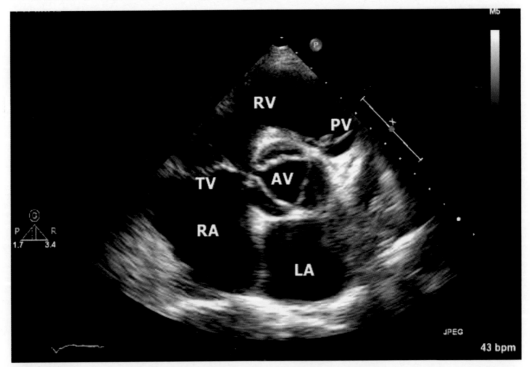

Figure 2.8a   TTE parasternal short axis view at the level of the aortic and pulmonic valve. AV, aortic valve; PV, pulmonic valve.

If you angle the head of the transducer slightly downward, you may see the bifurcation of the left main pulmonary artery into the right and left pulmonary arteries with the descending thoracic aorta just below it (Figure 2.8b). In this view, the distal portion of the aortic arch can be seen just below the bifurcation. Flow from a patent ductus arteriosus can often be visualized in this view (see also Figure 12.12b).

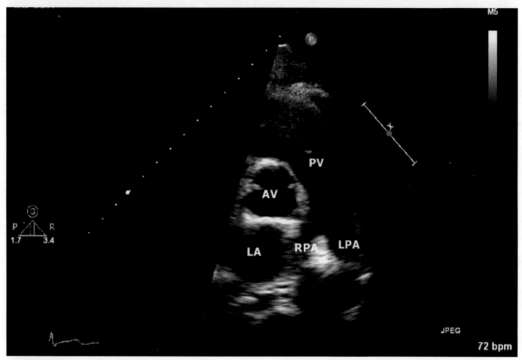

Figure 2.8b TTE parasternal short axis view showing the bifurcation of the pulmonary artery into the left pulmonary artery (LPA) and right pulmonary artery (RPA).

Identification of the aortic valve cusps: The normal aortic valve has three leaflets. Find the interatrial septum. When the valve is open, the noncoronary cusp intersects the interatrial septum. The right coronary cusp lies anterior (Figure 2.8c).

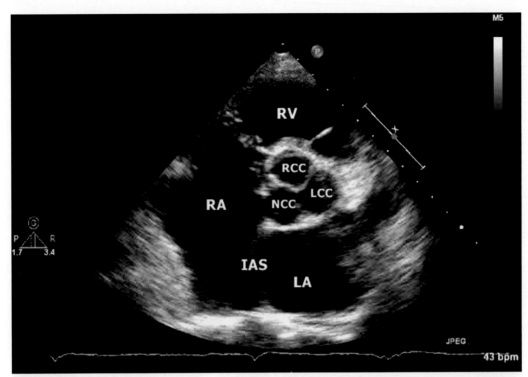

Figure 2.8c   TTE parasternal short axis view. The orientation of the three aortic valve cusps in relation to the interatrial septum (IAS). The noncoronary cusp (NCC) is bisected by the IAS, the right coronary cusp (RCC) lies anterior, and the left coronary cusp (LCC) lies posterior.

LEARNING DIRECTIVE

See Clip 2a.9: The same view showing diastolic right coronary artery flow at 3 o'clock along the aortic valve.

2.6   In the parasternal short axis view, the heart can be sliced like a loaf of bread to reveal multiple cross-sectional views. At the mitral valve level, both the anterior and posterior mitral valve leaflets are well seen (Figure 2.9a).

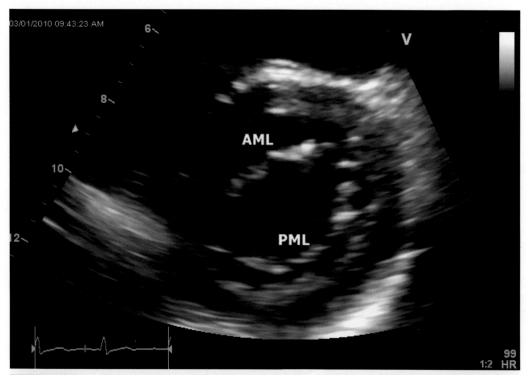

Figure 2.9a TTE parasternal short axis view at mitral valve level demonstrates the anterior mitral valve leaflet (AML) and posterior mitral valve leaflet (PML) in cross-section.

At papillary muscle level, both the posteromedial and anterolateral muscles are well seen in cross section (Figure 2.9b).

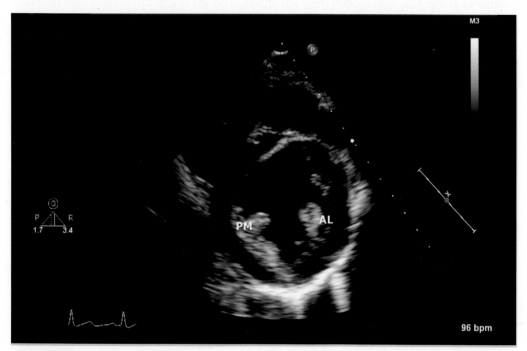

Figure 2.9b TEE parasternal short axis at the level of the papillary muscles. The anterolateral (AL) and posteromedial (PM) papillary muscles are well seen.

2.7   *Apical views* are obtained from or near the anteroaxillary line around the fifth or sixth intercostal space. The four-chamber view shows LA, RA, LV, RV, the mitral and tricuspid valves, and 7 of the 17 segments in the ASE wall motion map (for more details see also Chapter 15) (Figure 2.10).

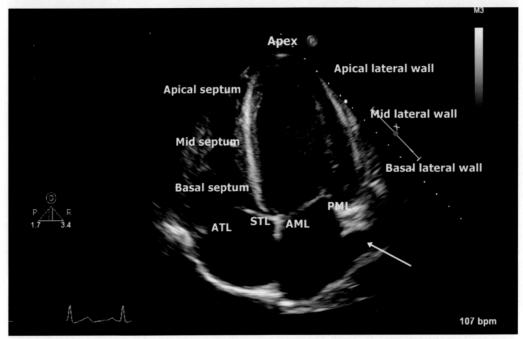

Figure 2.10   TTE apical four-chamber view. The anterior (AML) and posterior (PML) mitral valve leaflets, septal (STL) and anterior (ATL) tricuspid leaflets, and 7 of the 17 segments in the ASE wall motion map are shown. The left upper pulmonary vein (arrow) is also seen.

Rotating the transducer clockwise will produce the two-chamber view, which shows anterior and inferior LV walls as well as the mitral valve (Figure 2.11). Six more of the 17 segments of the ASE wall motion map are seen.

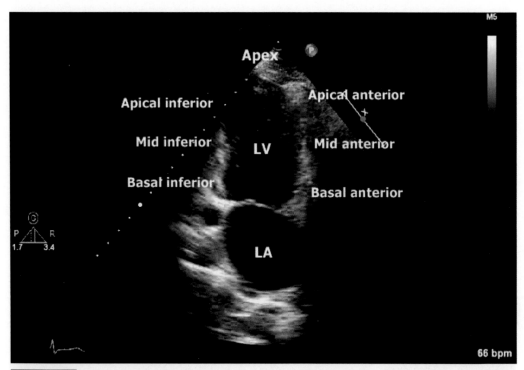

Figure 2.11   TTE apical two-chamber view describing the inferior and anterior LV walls. LA, left atrium.

Further clockwise rotation reveals the three-chamber view (Figure 2.12a), which includes the aortic valve as well as anterior septum and inferolateral wall.

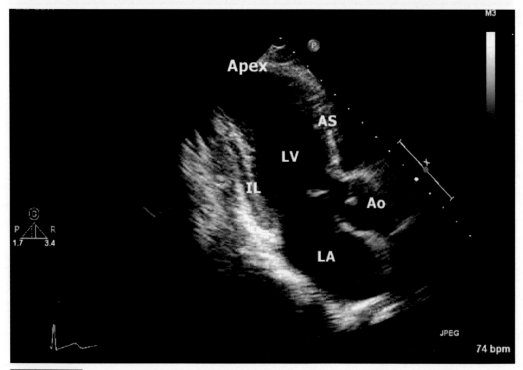

Figure 2.12a   TTE apical three-chamber long axis view. IL, inferolateral wall; AS, anteroseptal wall.

The five-chamber view also includes the aortic valve. In this view, the inferolateral and anteroseptal walls are seen (Figure 2.12b). Both five- and three-chamber views can be used for Doppler interrogation of the aortic valve and left ventricular outflow tract (LVOT).

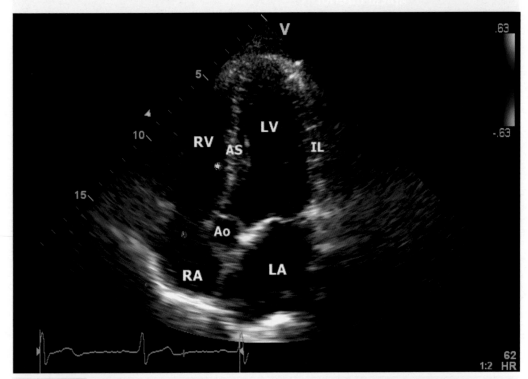

Figure 2.12b   TTE in the five-chamber view shows the inferolateral wall (IL) and anteroseptal wall (AS).

2.8   *Subcostal views* are obtained just to the left of the xiphoid process. They are most important in some patients for detection of an ASD, pericardial effusions, and estimation of RV size and systolic function (Figure 2.13a).

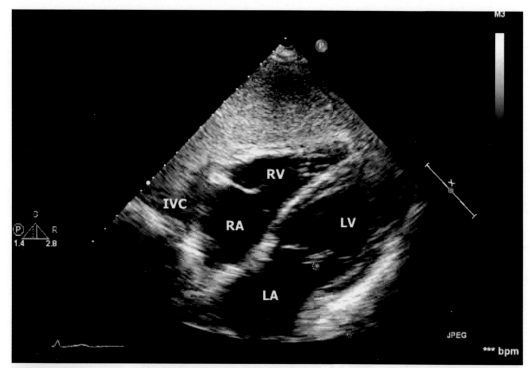

Figure 2.13a   TTE subcostal view in long axis shows all four cardiac chambers as well as the inferior vena cava (IVC).

A subcostal short axis view will show the great vessels in a configuration similar to the parasternal short axis view (Figure 2.13b).

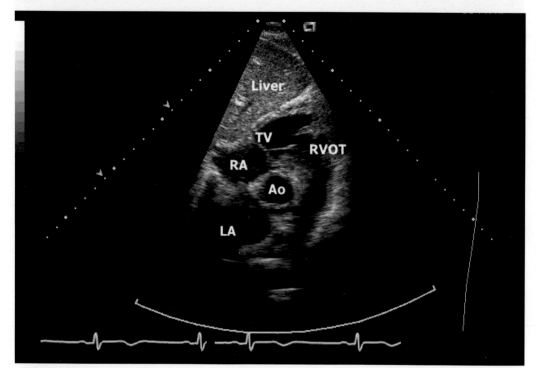

Figure 2.13b   TTE subcostal short axis view shows the LA, RA, and right ventricular outflow tract (RVOT), taken in systole with the tricuspid valve (TV) closed and the aortic (Ao) and pulmonic valves open and therefore not well visualized.

Tilting the transducer slightly medial will visualize the IVC and hepatic vein (Figure 2.13c). This view is critical for estimation of RA pressure and for evaluation of hepatic vein flow in the setting of constrictive pericarditis.

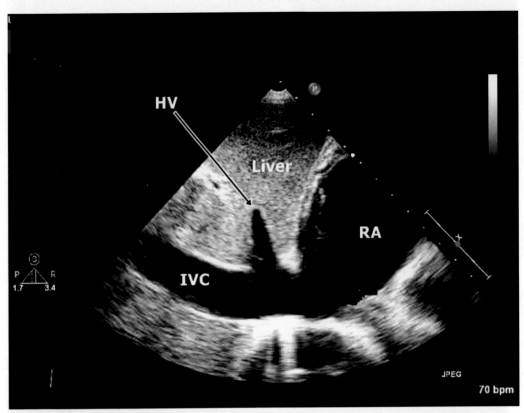

Figure 2.13c   TTE subcostal view. The hepatic vein (HV) can be seen entering the inferior vena cava (IVC).

Right-sided pleural effusions can also be seen in this view (Figure 2.13d).

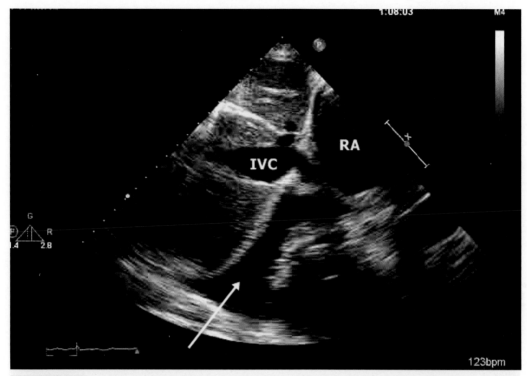

Figure 2.13d   TTE subcostal view. A large right-sided pleural effusion is well seen in the subcostal view (arrow).

Each of these locations provides multiple planes of view: long and short axis views for parasternals; two-, three-, four-, and five-chamber views for apicals; and long and short axis for subcostal views, as demonstrated in Figure 2.14.

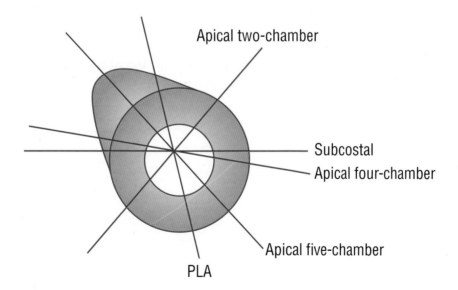

Figure 2.14   A schematic of the TTE parasternal short axis demonstrating the rotation of views through 360°. PLA, parasternal long axis.

2.9 *Suprasternal views*: From the suprasternal notch, the aortic arch and the left carotid and left subclavian arteries can be viewed. The *right pulmonary artery* is seen in cross section underneath the arch (Figure 2.15a).

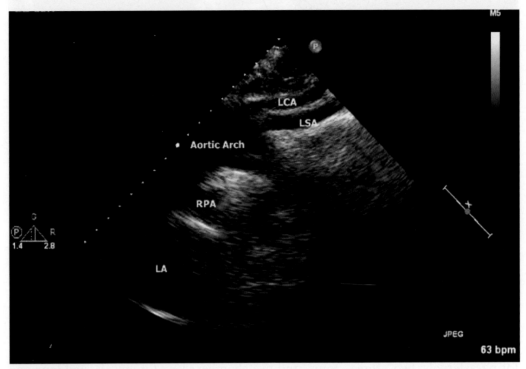

Figure 2.15a   TTE suprasternal view of the transverse aortic arch, left carotid artery (LCA), and left subclavian artery (LSA). The right pulmonary artery (RPA) passes beneath the arch, and the LA is inferior.

2.10   If the neck is extended slightly and the transducer is angled posteriorly, all four pulmonary veins can be seen in cross section at the top of the LA in what is colloquially called the "crab view" (Figure 2.15b).

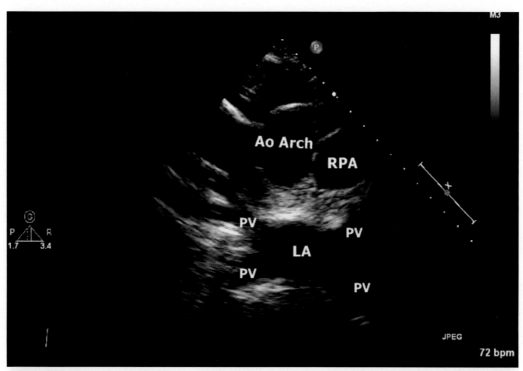

Figure 2.15b   TTE view from the suprasternal notch showing all four pulmonary veins (PV).

2.11   We often do not think about the pulmonary veins, but echocardiography reveals a great deal about their location and function. Three of the four *pulmonary veins* (left upper, left lower, and right upper) can often be seen in a typical four-chamber view (Figure 2.16a).

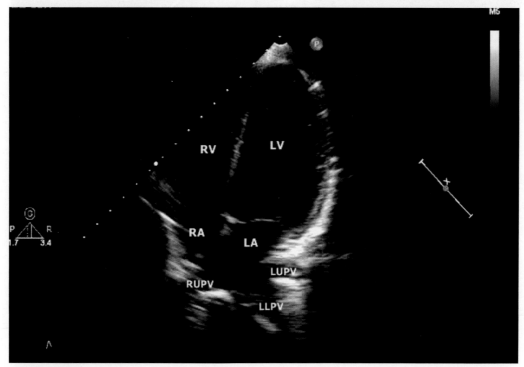

Figure 2.16a   TTE apical four-chamber view. The right upper pulmonary vein (RUPV), left upper pulmonary vein (LUPV), and left lower pulmonary vein (LLPV) can be seen.

LEARNING DIRECTIVE

See Clip 2a.18: Normal flow from the right upper pulmonary vein.

Flow from the left upper pulmonary vein can occasionally be seen and should be distinguished from mitral regurgitation by both its location and velocity (Figure 2.16b).

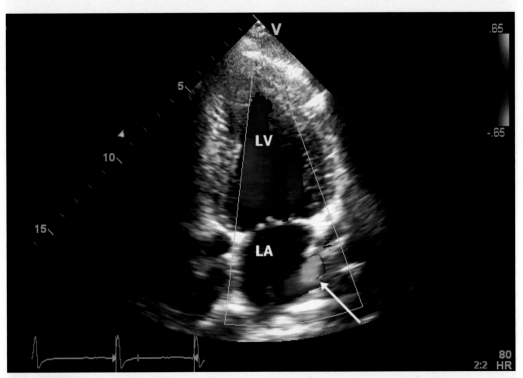

Figure 2.16b   TTE four-chamber view. Left upper pulmonary vein flow (arrow).

2.12 *TTE suprasternal view*: The brachiocephalic vein can often be seen in the suprasternal view (Figure 2.17).

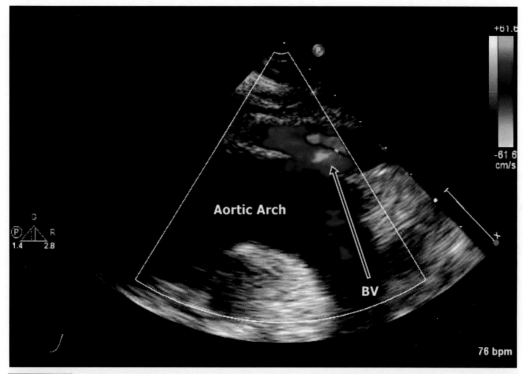

Figure 2.17   TTE suprasternal view. The brachiocephalic vein (BV; arrow) lies superior to the transverse aortic arch.

LEARNING DIRECTIVE

See Clip 2a.30: Normal-color Doppler flow through the brachiocephalic vein. Note the direction of flow is opposite to the arch just below.

2.13   The SVC in long axis is seen from the right suprasternal notch (Figure 2.18).

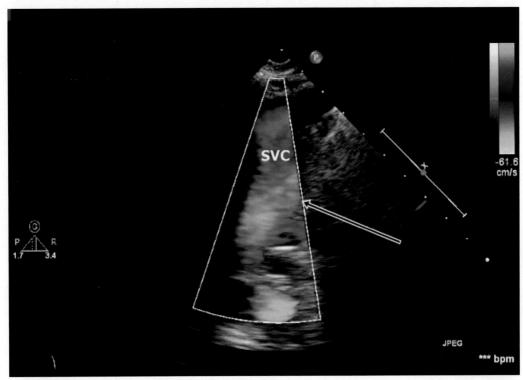

Figure 2.18 TTE right suprasternal notch view. The superior vena cava (SVC; arrow) can be seen in long axis from the right suprasternal notch.

LEARNING DIRECTIVE

See Clip 2a.32: Color flow through the SVC in the same view.

ADVANCED QUESTIONS

Q2.4 Which view demonstrates all four pulmonary veins simultaneously?

a. TEE midesophageal at 45° along the left atrial floor

b. TEE midesophageal view at 135°

c. TTE subcostal short axis with anterior angulation

d. TTE suprasternal view with posterior angulation

e. None of the above

Q2.5 Which view demonstrates right pleural effusions?

a. Parasternal long axis

b. Parasternal short axis

c. Apical four-chamber

d. Apical two-chamber

e. Subcostal

Q2.6 Where should the transducer be placed to demonstrate the SVC?

a. Second intercostal space to the left of the sternum

b. Second intercostal space to the right of the sternum

c. Left supraclavicular fossa

d. Right supraclavicular fossa

e. Subxiphoid notch

Q2.7   Where is the transducer located relative to proper position in the parasternal long axis image shown in Figure Q2.7?

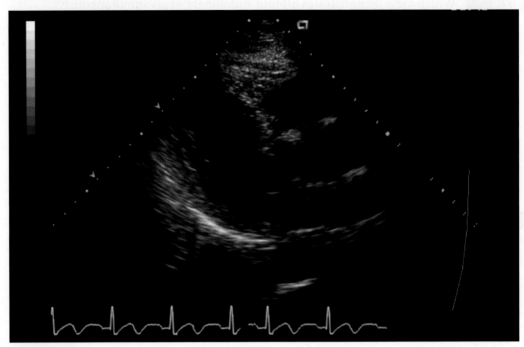

Figure Q2.7

    a. One interspace below the proper interspace

    b. One interspace above the proper interspace

    c. In the proper interspace but 2 cm lateral to the proper position

    d. In the proper interspace but 2 cm medial to the proper position

    e. The transducer is in the proper location.

Q2.8   The transverse pericardial sinus:

    a. Runs between the posterior LA wall and the ascending aorta

    b. Runs between the atrioventricular groove and the coronary sinus

    c. Runs between the aortic root and the main pulmonary artery

    d. Runs between the RA and the IVC

    e. Cannot be visualized by echocardiography

Q2.9   Which pulmonary vein is not visualized in the apical four-chamber view?

  a.   Left upper pulmonary vein

  b.   Left lower pulmonary vein

  c.   Right upper pulmonary vein

  d.   Right lower pulmonary vein

  e.   All four veins are seen.

Q2.10   Which of the following dimensions are typically measured at end-systole?

  a.   SWT and LV end-systolic dimension

  b.   LA dimension and LV end-systolic dimension

  c.   Aortic root dimension and LV end-systolic dimension

  d.   Septal wall thickness and pressure half-time

  e.   LV mass and pulmonary artery pressure

For Questions 2.11 and 2.12, refer to Figure Q2.11, which is obtained from the parasternal short axis view.

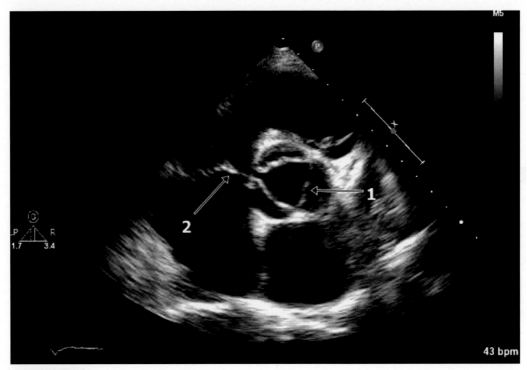

Figure Q2.11

Q2.11   To which structure is arrow 1 pointing?

    a.   Right coronary leaflet of the aortic valve

    b.   Left coronary leaflet of the aortic valve

    c.   Noncoronary leaflet of the aortic valve

    d.   More information is needed.

Q2.12   To which structure is arrow 2 pointing?

    a.   Anterior leaflet of the tricuspid valve

    b.   Septal leaflet of the tricuspid valve

    c.   Posterior leaflet of the tricuspid valve

    d.   None of the above

    e.   More information is needed.

Q2.13   Systolic function of the inferior LV wall segments is best visualized in what view?

    a.   Parasternal long axis

    b.   Apical four-chamber

    c.   Apical two-chamber

    d.   Apical three-chamber

    e.   Subcostal long axis

ANSWERS

Q2.4   d: Also known as the crab view, a name derived from the resemblance to a crab of all four pulmonary veins in cross section. (Section **2.10**)

Q2.5   e: Left-sided effusions are seen in multiple views adjacent to the inferolateral wall. Right-sided pleural effusions are best seen in the subcostal view. None of the apical views image the right chest with sufficient clarity to demonstrate a right-sided pleural effusion. (Section **2.3b**)

Q2.6   d: See Section **2.13**.

Q2.7   a: Placing the transducer in a lower interspace (a maneuver sometimes necessary to produce a quality image) will tilt the apex toward the top of the screen. (Section **2.1**)

Q2.8   a: The transverse sinus provides a potential (and usually empty) space between the LA and the aortic root. When fluid is present, the sinus can also be seen by TEE in a 90° view of the aortic valve and root. (Section **2.10**)

Q2.9   d: The right lower pulmonary vein is too posterior to be seen in this view. The right lower pulmonary vein can be seen by TEE at 40–60° in a high-midesophageal view of the LA and aortic root. (Section **2.11**)

Q2.10   b: See Section **2.1**.

Q2.11   b: The noncoronary leaflet is bisected by the interatrial septum. The right coronary leaflet is anterior to the noncoronary leaflet. (Section **2.5**)

Q2.12   b: The posterior tricuspid leaflet is only seen in the RV inflow view or in the subcostal short axis view if the valve is well visualized. In every other conventional view, the septal tricuspid leaflet is either directly attached to the septum or is adjacent to the aortic root. (Section **2.5**)

Q2.13   c: See Section **2.7**.

3 DOPPLER ECHOCARDIOGRAPHY

Q3.1 The Doppler frequency shift is:

    a. Directly proportional to the speed of the sound source and inversely proportional to the propagation speed of sound in the medium

    b. Inversely proportional to the speed of the sound source and directly proportional to the propagation speed of sound in the medium

    c. Directly proportional to the speed of the sound source and directly proportional to the propagation speed of sound in the medium

    d. Inversely proportional to the speed of the sound source and inversely proportional to the propagation speed of sound in the medium

Q3.2 Which of the following combinations will produce aliasing of a pulsed Doppler signal?

    a. The magnitude of the observed frequency shift is less than one-half of the transducer frequency.

    b. The magnitude of the observed frequency shift in the signal is less than one-half of the PRF.

    c. The magnitude of the observed frequency shift in the signal is equal to the PRF.

    d. The magnitude of the observed frequency shift is zero.

    e. The magnitude of the observed frequency shift in the signal is greater than twice the PRF.

Q3.3   In a patient with aortic stenosis, the peak transvalvular flow velocity is 4 m/sec and the peak subvalvular (LVOT) velocity is 2 m/sec. The peak calculated aortic valve gradient is:

a.   64 mm Hg

b.   60 mm Hg

c.   48 mm Hg

d.   16 mm Hg

The Doppler Equation

3.1   The Doppler equation describes the relationship between the shift in frequency (Δf) that a moving sound source (or a sound wave reflected off a moving object) produces and the speed with which it is moving.

In the equation that follows:

- f_0 = transmitted frequency

- $\cos\theta$ = the angle at which the sound source reflects off the moving object

- v = the speed of the object

- c = the speed of the ultrasound in the medium

$$f = f_1 - f_0 = \Delta f$$
$$= \frac{(2f_0)(\cos\theta)(v)}{c}$$

The equation can be manipulated algebraically to solve for velocity (v), which is what makes Doppler imaging so powerful:

$$v = \frac{(c)(\Delta f)}{(2f_0)(\cos\theta)}$$

3.2   Because $\cos\theta$ is in the denominator, the more parallel the Doppler beam is with flow, the more accurate will be the frequency that is measured, considering that the cosine of $0° = 1$. By contrast, if the transducer is perpendicular to flow, you will see no frequency shift at all, as the cosine of $90° = 0$. By convention, the frequency shift is displayed as positive when the flow is moving toward the transducer and negative when moving away. Even though cardiac ultrasound occurs at frequencies well above audible (20 kHz), the shift itself is well within the audible range (0–20 kHz). That audible shift is the sound you hear when the sonographer is producing a spectral Doppler tracing.

3.3   Doppler comes in two forms, *pulse wave* (PW) and *continuous wave* (CW). With PW Doppler, the transducer sends a pulse, waits for the pulse to return, and then sends another pulse. Because the time from the transmission of the pulse to its return is known, PW Doppler can spatially locate the flow from which it reflects. However, the ability of PW Doppler to sample higher velocity frequencies is limited by the PRF (more on this in a moment).

With CW Doppler, one transducer is sending while the other is receiving simultaneously. Under these conditions, only the frequency shift is measured, and the spatial location of the reflecting flow cannot be established. Because there is no PRF, there is no maximum limit to the velocity of the flow that can be interrogated. CW Doppler can only be displayed using a spectral display. PW Doppler can be displayed using either spectral display or color display.

3.4   Both forms of Doppler actually send out a number of scan lines and produce a spectrum of frequency shifts from red cells traveling at different velocities and in different locations. The total region scanned comprises the *sample volume*. Somehow, the differing frequency shifts from all the pulses must be reconciled. Spectral Doppler display uses a *fast Fourier transformation* summation algorithm that assigns a value for both location and intensity to each frequency shift to allow for its proper location to be displayed within the resultant image. For color display, phases of those waves most similar are summed together by *autocorrelation* to produce a single coherent output.

3.5   *Aliasing* occurs when the *sampling frequency falls below the level of the frequency shift* (and therefore the velocity) of the moving object being sampled. This phenomenon is common to any sampling system. Think, for example, of the spinning wagon wheel in the movies. The wheel is rotating at hundreds of revolutions/min, yet the sampling rate of movie film is only 30/sec. The spokes of the wheel are no longer visible, and all you perceive is the blur produced by the inadequate sampling rate. In PW Doppler, the sampling frequency is represented by the PRF. The frequency shift at which aliasing occurs is called the *Nyquist limit* and is defined as one-half of the PRF.

Figure 3.1 illustrates the limits of sampling. Both waves are sampled at the same sampling frequency, but the results of each sampling will look quite different. Because of aliasing, the sampling device cannot reliably identify the wave with the higher frequency, as each sampling occurs during a different point in the phase of the wave. The wide, low-frequency wave will be sampled accurately; the narrow, high-frequency wave will not.

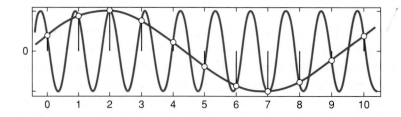

Figure 3.1   The effect of sampling rate upon proper identification of the waveform.

Thus, the spectral Doppler tracing at this PRF will produce a picture that has a false identity, which is what the word alias means.

3.6   *To avoid aliasing:*

1. Raise (or lower) the baseline.

2. Decrease the imaging depth.

3. Raise the PRF.

4. Lower the frequency of the transducer.

5. Decrease the size of the sample volume.

In general, most spectral Doppler signals will alias at frequency shifts that produce velocities > 2 m/sec, and color Doppler signals will alias at velocities of > 0.7 m/sec.

3.7   Color-flow Doppler is a form of pulse Doppler and therefore obeys all the rules of pulse Doppler. Because the sample flow volume of color Doppler is usually large, its Nyquist limit tends to be relatively small. The key to the color map at the right-hand side of the screen in Figure 3.2 provides critical information.

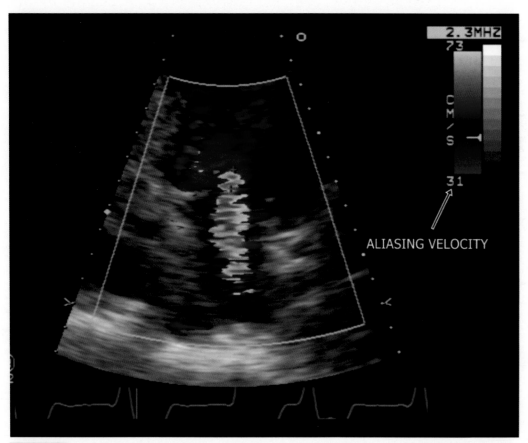

Figure 3.2   TTE apical two-chamber view in a patient with mitral regurgitation demonstrating the location of the aliasing velocity of the color Doppler signal (labeled arrow).

The numbers at the top right-hand side of the screen in Figure 3.2 represent the Nyquist limit of the Doppler signal in both directions. This value can be adjusted up or down. The change in color intensity, when displayed in a vertical fashion, represents the relation of color to velocity. This display is termed *velocity mode*. When the display intensity is graded horizontally, the map is displayed in *variance mode*. The color mosaic visible on the screen also provides a qualitative measure of *turbulence* or turbulent flow, which, when present, can provide an important clue to the presence of a variety of disease states.

3.8   The turbulence of a flow is best described by the *Reynolds number*. The Reynolds number is a dimensionless quantity defined as:

$$\text{Reynolds number} = \frac{\text{fluid velocity} \times \text{fluid density} \times \text{orifice diameter}}{\text{fluid viscosity}}$$

Increasing blood velocity, blood density, or the size of the hole through which the blood is moving will increase turbulence; increasing viscosity will decrease it. Reynolds numbers greater than 3000 are considered fully turbulent.

The Bernoulli Equation

3.9   The Bernoulli equation relates velocity of flow to the pressure gradient between the two chambers. It has three components: (1) convective acceleration, (2) flow acceleration, and (3) viscous friction:

$$p_1 - p_2 = \tfrac{1}{2}\rho(V_2^2 - V_1^2) \qquad\qquad (1)$$

$$+\rho_1 \int^2 \frac{dV}{dt}\,ds \qquad\qquad (2)$$

$$+R(V) \qquad\qquad (3)$$

Because flow acceleration is linear and viscous friction is minimal, these components can usually be ignored, and the equation simplifies to the convective component:

$$p_2 - p_1 = \tfrac{1}{2}\rho(V_2^2 - V_1^2)$$

In this equation:

- $p_2 - p_1 =$ the pressure gradient between the two locations that you measure

- $(V_2^2 - V_1^2) =$ the flow velocities at those two locations, V_2 and V_1

- $\rho =$ blood density (1.06 g/ml)

If V_1 is small (≤ 1 m/sec), you can ignore it.

Changing the constant by converting to mm Hg gives you:

$$\Delta P = 4V_2^2$$

If V_1 is > 1 m/sec, however, you should generally take it into account.

Calculating Stroke Volume Using the Velocity Time Integral and the Orifice Diameter

3.10 The *velocity time integral* (VTI) (Figure 3.3) is the area under the curve produced by a spectral Doppler flow. It describes total flow per unit of time. Because the time integral of velocity is distance, the VTI is measured in centimeters (cm).

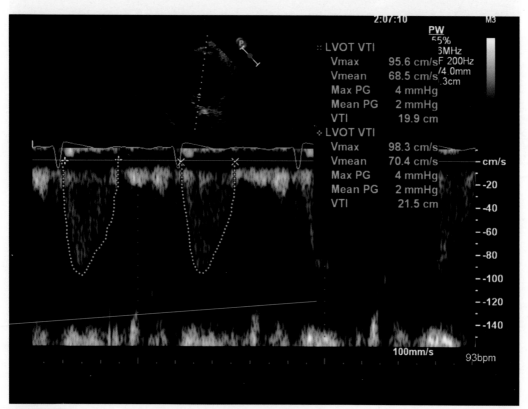

Figure 3.3 VTI in the LVOT measured by PW Doppler from the apical five-chamber view. The average of the two measurements is 20.7 cm.

The LVOT diameter (Figure 3.4) allows you to estimate the area through which the VTI is flowing.

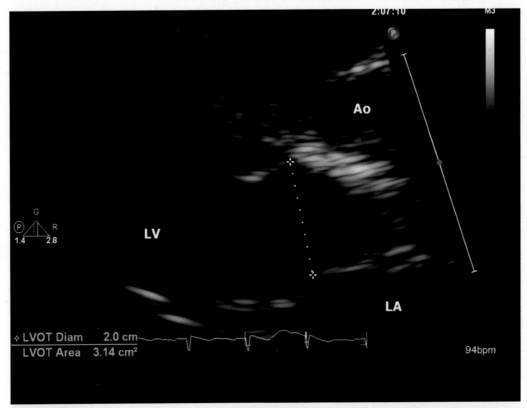

Figure 3.4   TTE parasternal long axis demonstrates the LVOT diameter.

To calculate the orifice area, assume the LVOT is circular and use the diameter (D) to calculate the area as:

$$\text{area} = 3.14(D/2)^2 = 0.785D^2$$

If you integrate three dimensions, you produce a volume as:

$$\text{LV stroke volume} = \text{LVOT flow} \times \text{LVOT area}$$
$$= \text{VTI} \times \text{LVOT area}$$

In the example shown in Figures 3.3 and 3.4, the stroke volume is:

$$\text{LV stroke volume} = 0.785 \times 2.0 \text{ cm}^2 \times 20.7 \text{ cm} = 65 \text{ cc}$$

As with any college physics problem, you must be careful with your units and your decimal places. If the VTI is shown in m/sec, you must convert the value to cm/sec so the units match. One can also appreciate that errors in the LVOT diameter are magnified because the term is squared. Thus, a 10% error in VTI will produce a 10% error in stroke volume, while a 10% error in diameter (0.9–1.1) will produce a 19–21% error (0.9² to 1.1²) in stroke volume.

3.11 You can use a spectral Doppler VTI to quantify any *flow volume across an orifice*. You will use this concept again and again when it comes to quantification of valvular regurgitation, because you can quantify regurgitation by subtracting the stroke volume of the regurgitant valve from the non-regurgitant valve. If you know the heart rate (HR), you can also use this calculation to estimate cardiac output:

$$\text{cardiac output} = \text{stroke volume} \times \text{HR}$$

Use of Doppler for Assessment of Pressure Gradients Across an Orifice

3.12 The spectral Doppler jet quantifies the pressure gradient across the orifice. If you know (or can reasonably guess) the pressure gradient on one side of the orifice, you can add (or subtract) the gradient to determine the pressure on the other side. This means that any regurgitant jet can be used to gauge the pressure on one side of it as follows:

Pulmonary artery (PA) systolic pressure = 4(peak tricuspid regurgitant jet velocity)² + estimated RA pressure

PA diastolic pressure = 4(end-diastolic pulmonary regurgitation velocity)² + estimated RV end-diastolic pressure

LA pressure = systolic blood pressure – 4(peak mitral regurgitation velocity)²

LV end-diastolic pressure = aortic diastolic blood pressure – 4(end-diastolic aortic regurgitation jet velocity)²

and even:

RV systolic pressure = systemic systolic blood pressure – 4(ventricular septal defect jet velocity)²

Suppose, for example, that the peak mitral regurgitation jet in a patient with mild mitral regurgitation is 5 m/sec:

$$\text{peak gradient} = 4(5 \text{ m/sec})^2 = 100 \text{ mm Hg}$$

(This is not surprising, by the way, since even mild mitral regurgitation will produce a gradient that reflects the pressure difference between the LV and LA in systole, which is almost always large.) If the systolic blood pressure is 120 mm Hg, then the LA systolic pressure can be estimated as:

$$120 \text{ mm Hg} - 100 \text{ mm Hg} = 20 \text{ mm Hg}$$

A word of caution is order. Because the velocity is squared, a 10% error in the velocity will again lead to a 19–21% error in the calculated pressure gradient, a value that can lead to large practical errors in estimated pressures.

ADVANCED QUESTIONS

Q3.4   Which of the following maneuvers will avoid aliasing of a Doppler signal?

   a.   Decreasing the PRF

   b.   Increasing the sample depth

   c.   Decreasing the sample volume

   d.   Switching from CW Doppler to PW Doppler

   e.   Increasing the transducer frequency

Q3.5   An increase in which of the following factors will produce a decrease in turbulence?

   a.   Blood velocity

   b.   Blood viscosity

   c.   Blood density

   d.   Blood temperature

   e.   Orifice diameter

Q3.6   The patient's blood pressure is 135/40 mm Hg. The LV end-diastolic pressure, as calculated from the information provided in the transaortic CW Doppler tracing in Figure Q3.6, is:

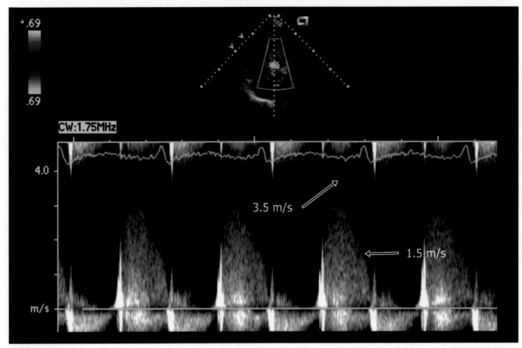

Figure Q3.6

    a.   5 mm Hg

    b.   15 mm Hg

    c.   25 mm Hg

    d.   31 mm Hg

    e.   35 mm Hg

Q3.7   The IVC in the patient whose spectral Doppler tracing is shown in Figure
Q3.7 measures 2 cm in diameter and collapses less than 50% with respiration. The estimated pulmonary artery diastolic pressure is:

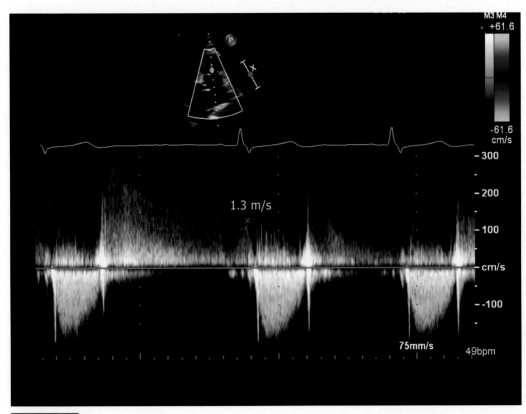

Figure Q3.7

    a.   < 6 mm Hg

    b.   6–10 mm Hg

    c.   10–15 mm Hg

    d.   15–20 mm Hg

    e.   > 20 mm Hg

Q3.8   Which parameter is a measure of increasing turbulent flow detectable by Doppler interrogation?

a. Increasing fluid velocity

b. Decreasing fluid density

c. Decreasing orifice radius

d. Increasing fluid viscosity

e. Increasing lumen length

ANSWERS

Q3.4   c: All of the listed parameters affect aliasing, but all the other choices will *increase* its likelihood. (Sections **3.5** and **3.6**)

Q3.5   b: Turbulence is directly proportional to flow velocity, fluid density, and orifice diameter; it is inversely proportional to fluid viscosity, so increasing viscosity will decrease turbulence (i.e., make the Reynolds number smaller). This is admittedly an obscure question and deliberately worded in a rather tortuous fashion. (Section **3.8**)

Q3.6   d

$$\text{LVEDP} = \text{LV end-diastolic blood pressure} - \text{aortic regurgitation pressure gradient at end-diastole}$$

From Figure Q3.6:

$$40 \text{ mm Hg} - 4(1.5 \text{ cm})^2 = 40 - 9 = 31 \text{ mm Hg}$$

Note that the pressure value that is used is at the end of diastole. (Section **3.12**)

Q3.7   e

$$\text{PA diastolic pressure} = \text{RA pressure} + \text{pulmonic regurgitant velocity } t \text{ at end-diastole}$$

From Figure Q3.7:

$$15 \text{ mm Hg (from the noncollapsing IVC)} + 4(1.3)^2$$
$$= 15 + 5.2 = 20.2 \text{ mm Hg}$$

(Section **3.12**)

Q3.8   a: See Question 3.2 and Section 3.8.

4 TRANSESOPHAGEAL ECHOCARDIOGRAPHY

Q4.1 Which of the following is a well-described complication of TEE?

   a. Soft palate perforation

   b. Laryngeal perforation

   c. Pharyngeal perforation

   d. Tracheal perforation

   e. Intestinal perforation

Q4.2 Which of the following conditions is an absolute contraindication to TEE?

   a. Dysphagia

   b. Esophageal diverticulum

   c. Obstructive sleep apnea

   d. Esophageal varices

   e. Septic shock

Q4.3 Which structure is least well seen by TEE?

   a. Posterior tricuspid leaflet

   b. RV free wall

   c. Left circumflex coronary artery

   d. Right pulmonary artery

   e. Left lower pulmonary vein

ANSWERS: 4.1. c; 4.2. b; 4.3. b

4.1 While TEE provides a unique tool for the evaluation of cardiac structures, as with any test, it comes with its own set of caveats and complications. It is extraordinarily useful for visualization of posterior structures, especially the mitral valve, LA, interatrial septum, and pulmonary veins, but it is less helpful for evaluation of anterior structures such as the free wall of the RV and the pulmonic valve. It is a moderately invasive test that usually employs conscious sedation, can be uncomfortable for patients, and has a known (albeit small) complication rate. Because its views are narrowly fixed, the position of the heart within the mediastinum will affect both what you can see and how well you can see it. Vertically oriented (straight up and down) hearts will produce excellent views reminiscent of four-chamber views by TTE, in which the LV apex is well seen and the RV is nicely laid out. More horizontally positioned hearts will be more challenging to image, because every view assumes some form of a cross-sectional aspect, and the transition from midesophageal to midgastric views can be quite abrupt.

4.2 In contrast to TTE, the posterior position of the probe rotates the vertical orientation of view 180°. In effect, you are looking from above and behind the heart in cross-sectional views, so that posterior structures appear at the top of the screen and anterior structures are at the bottom. Left-to-right orientation is unchanged compared to TTE.

4.3 Every TEE should be preceded by a brief patient evaluation that confirms the appropriateness of the study, including a formal history and review of past medical history, with special care to ensure that no contraindications to the procedure are present (see Appendix B). Absolute contraindications include severe esophageal disease such as proximal tumor, stricture, or proximal Zenker (esophageal) diverticulum. Relative contraindications to TEE (or conditions that at least deserve further investigation prior to the procedure) include a history of dysphasia or odynophagia, esophageal varicies, or undiagnosed upper gastrointestinal bleeding. The most feared complication, esophageal perforation, is quite rare, with a rate of less than 1:1000 cases, and is more common in the setting of the previously cited conditions. Probe overheating may also occur, especially with the new three-dimensional (3D) probes, although in the current era, most TEE probes will automatically shut down before reaching a temperature that places the esophagus at risk for thermal injury (42°C). Conditions that complicate the use of conscious sedation, such as heart failure, pulmonary disease, or obstructive sleep apnea, should be defined, and the need for anesthesiologist assistance should be determined. Patients should be made NPO (nothing by mouth) for 4–6 hours prior to the procedure. The pharynx is anesthetized either by gargling with a topical anesthetic solution or by direct application of anesthetic gel. Gag reflex should be well suppressed prior to esophageal intubation.

4.4 A multiplane TEE probe provides four different types of manipulations for probe placement and obtaining of a particular view: (1) Proximal-distal position within the esophagus, (2) rotation of the probe head by rotating the handle, (3) anti-flexion, retroflexion, and lateral rotation of the probe head using the two knobs provided in the handle, and (4) changing the plane of view using the multiplane feature (usually two buttons on the handle). In general, a sequential approach to each view is taken: First, the appropriate level within the esophagus is reached. Next, the proper view is obtained through a combination of probe rotation and probe flexion. Last, a series of planes across the entire 180° are obtained and recorded. For a more comprehensive guide to a TEE study the reader is referred to Kothavale A, Yeon SB, Manning WJ. A systematic approach to performing a comprehensive transesophageal echocardiogram: A call to order. *BMC Cardiovascular Disorders* 2009;9:18.

Normal Transesophageal Views

4.5   *Midesophageal views*: These views provide an excellent look at the LV in a longitudinal orientation (Figure 4.1), as well as both the mitral leaflets and the LV and RV inflow tracts.

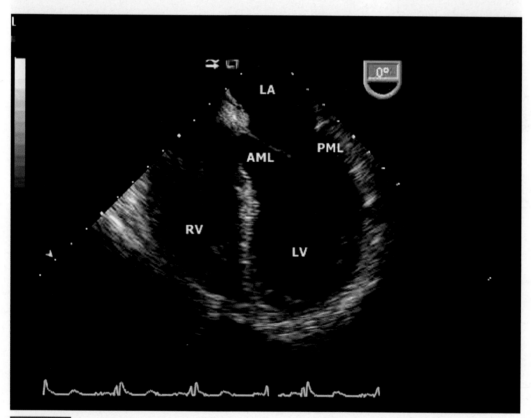

Figure 4.1   TEE four-chamber midesophageal view. AML, anterior mitral leaflet; PML, posterior mitral leaflet.

If the probe is withdrawn, the aortic valve will come directly into view and can be interrogated through 180°. Vertical views (45–75°) (Figure 4.2) will provide cross-sectional views of the aortic valve and allow identification of its leaflets.

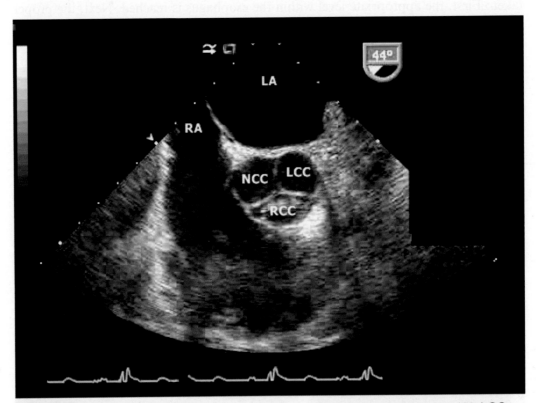

Figure 4.2   TEE midesophageal view of the aortic valve in cross section at ~45°. LCC, left coronary cusp; NCC, noncoronary cusp; RCC, right coronary cusp.

From about 100° onward, the aortic root and ascending aorta can be well seen (Figure 4.3).

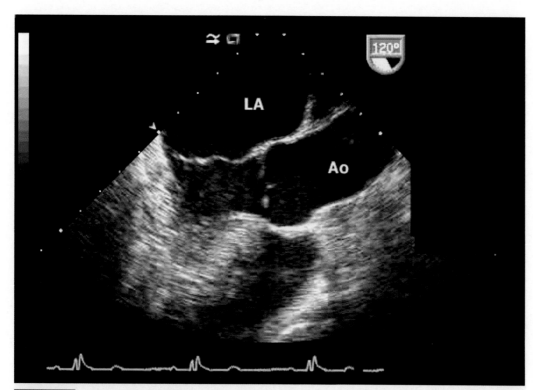

Figure 4.3   TEE midesophageal view. The LVOT, aortic root, and ascending aorta (Ao) are best seen between 120° and 135°.

As with TTE aortic views, the noncoronary cusp is bifurcated by the septum, the right coronary cusp is anterior (toward the bottom of the screen), and the left coronary cusp is superior.

The left main coronary artery can usually be identified (Figure 4.4).

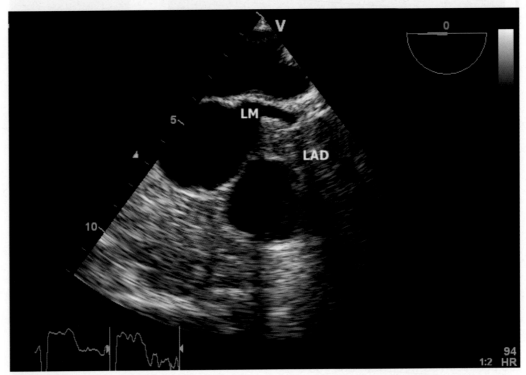

Figure 4.4   TEE midesophageal view. The left main coronary artery (LM) is readily seen.

LEARNING DIRECTIVE

See Clip 4.21: A still frame in the midesophagus shows the left main bifurcation.

4.6   The left atrial appendage is well seen at the midesophageal level by placing the mitral valve in the center of the screen, withdrawing slightly until the valve disappears, and providing maximum antiflexion (Figure 4.5). The left upper pulmonary vein is also seen in this view. From 45°, the probe at the level of the aortic valve, the probe can be rotated counterclockwise to reveal the right upper and lower pulmonary veins (Figure 4.6).

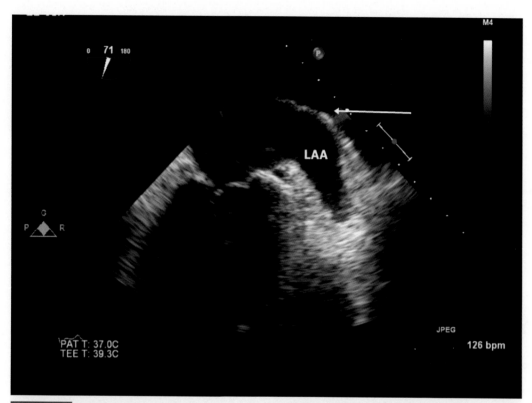

Figure 4.5   TEE midesophageal view. Left atrial appendage (LAA) and left upper pulmonary vein (arrow).

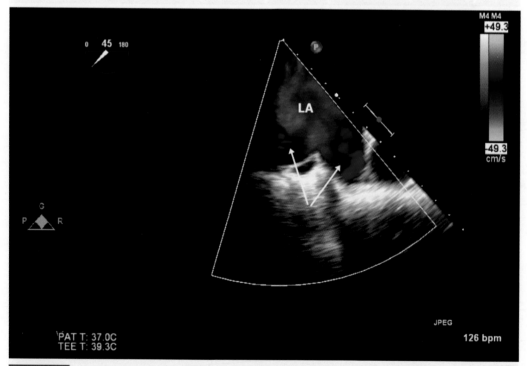

Figure 4.6   TEE midesophageal view. The right pulmonary veins (arrows).

4.7   *Right-sided views* are obtained by rotating the probe head clockwise and revealing the RA, interatrial septum, and septal and anterior tricuspid leaflets (Figure 4.7). Rotating the plane of view further, between 90° and 135°, will produce a bicaval view in which the superior vena cava is on the left of the screen and the inferior vena cava is on the right (Figure 4.8).

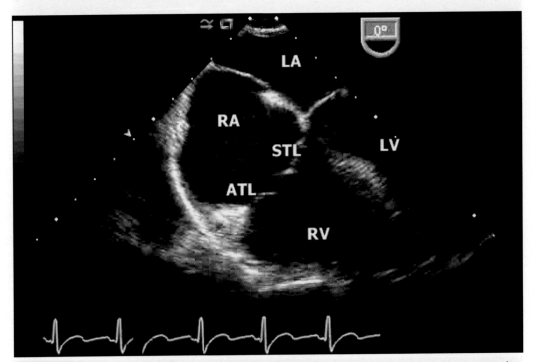

Figure 4.7   TEE lower esophageal view showing the RA and intra-atrial septum, anterior tricuspid leaflet (ATL) and septal tricuspid leaflet (STL).

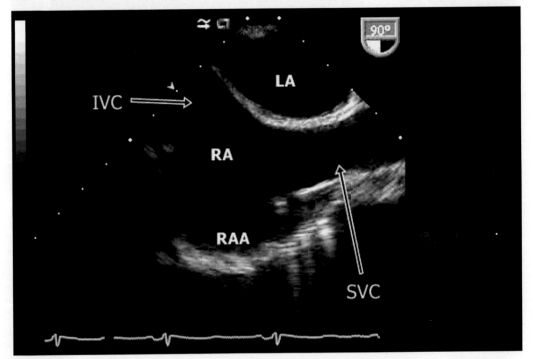

Figure 4.8   TEE midesophageal bicaval view. IVC, inferior vena cava; RAA, right atrial appendage; SVC, superior vena cava.

4.8 *Midgastric views* are found by placing the LV in the center of the screen, advancing the probe further through the gastroesophageal junction, and providing antiflexion to provide maximum contact in the fundus of the stomach. At 0°, the LV can be well seen in cross section; this view provides the best approximation of LV systolic function (Figure 4.9a). Vertical views lay out the LV along its axis and allow for visualization of the mitral valve (Figure 4.9b).

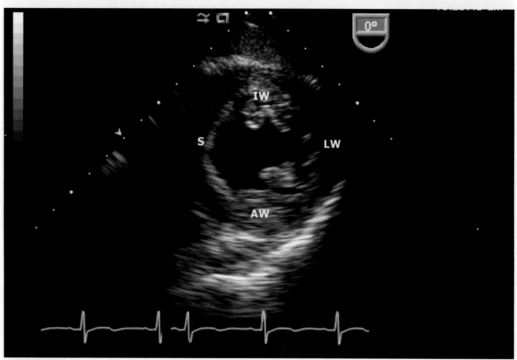

Figure 4.9a   TTE midgastric view at papillary muscle level. AW, anterior wall; IW, inferior wall; LW, lateral wall; S, septum.

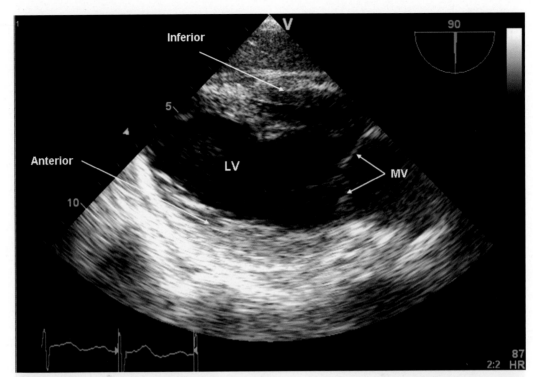

Figure 4.9b   TEE midgastric view of the LV at 90°. The inferior wall lies at the top of the screen. The anterior wall lies at the bottom.

4.9   *Deep-gastric views* can be obtained by a combination of further probe advancement followed by maximal insertion and flexion (Figure 4.10). This view alone allows for direct inline interrogation of the LVOT and therefore provides information necessary for estimation of aortic valve area using the continuity equation. LVOT diameter is obtained at the midesophageal level anywhere from 120° to 135°.

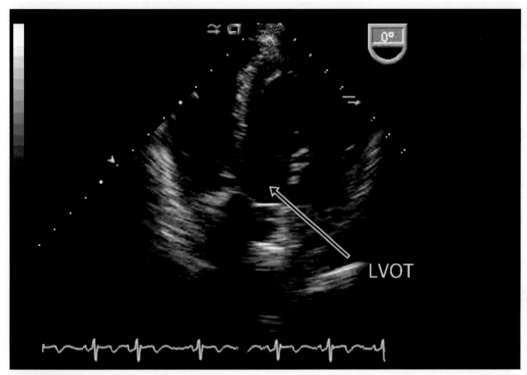

Figure 4.10   TEE deep-gastric view showing the left ventricular outflow tract (LVOT, arrow) and aortic valve in long axis.

4.10   A typical study is completed by directing the probe posteriorly in the horizontal orientation (0°) and visualizing the descending thoracic aorta in cross section while withdrawing the probe (Figure 4.11). These views allow for detection of aortic disease, especially atheroma, aneurysm, and descending aortic dissection.

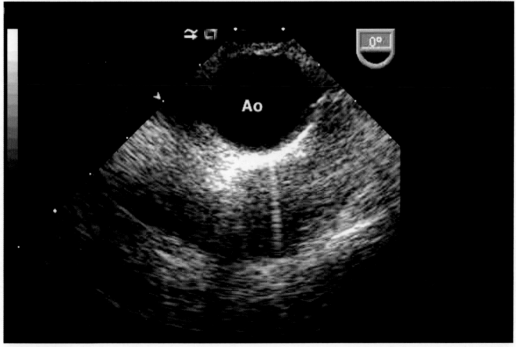

Figure 4.11   TEE midesophageal view showing the descending aorta (Ao) in cross-section.

ADVANCED QUESTIONS

Q4.4   At what angle are both the inferior vena cava and superior vena cava best visualized simultaneously by TEE?

a.   0–30°

b.   30–45°

c.   45–75°

d.   75–115°

e.   150–180°

Q4.5   You are performing an elective TEE when you notice the probe temperature rising to 42°C. At this point you should:

a.   Continue the study after infusing cooled saline intravenously.

b.   Turn off the 3D and color-flow Doppler and wait for the probe to cool to 37°C.

c.   Immediately remove the probe.

d.   Continue the study without further interruption.

Q4.6   In patients with tricuspid, aortic valve, and mitral valve replacements, which valve leads to shadows or interferes with visualization of the other?

a.   Aortic interferes with mitral.

b.   Mitral interferes with aortic.

c.   Tricuspid interferes with aortic.

d.   Tricuspid interferes with mitral.

e.   There is no interference for any valve.

Q4.7 Which TEE views allow for direct estimation of aortic valve area using 2D measurement?

a. High esophageal

b. Midesophageal

c. Midgastric

d. Transgastric

e. Deep gastric

Q4.8 Which TEE views are required for estimation of aortic valve area using the continuity equation?

a. Midesophageal and midgastric

b. Midesophageal and deep gastric

c. Midgastric and deep gastric

d. Bicaval and midgastric

e. Aortic valve area by TEE cannot be estimated by direct planimetry.

ANSWERS

Q4.4   d: This is the range of plane angulation in which the bicaval view is best visualized. (Section **4.7**)

Q4.5   b: Turning off the 3D and color Doppler would decrease the energy. (Section **4.3**)

Q4.6   b: The posterior location of the mitral valve prosthesis will often produce one or more acoustic shadows that obscure the aortic valve. (Section **4.1**)

Q4.7   b: Direct planimetry of the aortic valve area in cross section in the midesophageal view has been validated. (Section **4.9**)

Q4.8   b: The midesophageal view allows for measurement of the LVOT diameter, and the deep-gastric view allows for measurement of the LVOT and atrioventricular VTIs. (Sections **4.4** and **4.9**)

5

TISSUE DOPPLER AND STRAIN IMAGING

PRACTICE QUESTIONS

Q5.1 Which of the following relations defines strain rate?

    a. Change in myocardial segment length divided by initial length

    b. Peak velocity of a myocardial segment divided by time

    c. The sum of isovolumic relaxation time and isovolumic contraction time, divided by ejection time

    d. Chamber diameter divided by wall thickness

    e. Change in myocardial strain with time

Q5.2 Which is the *most* sensitive measure for detection of myocardial ischemia during dobutamine infusion?

    a. ST depression

    b. Left ventricular dilatation

    c. New abnormal wall motion

    d. Decrease in systolic strain

    e. Decrease in postsystolic shortening

Q5.3 Tissue doppler imaging (TDI) measures:

    a. High-velocity, high-amplitude signals

    b. Low-velocity, low-amplitude signals

    c. High-velocity, low-amplitude signals

    d. Low-velocity, high-amplitude signals

    e. None of the above

5.1 As with standard Doppler, tissue Doppler imaging (TDI) measures the frequency shift produced by reflecting a sound wave off a moving object. In the case of TDI, the object is myocardial tissue itself. The major difference between TDI and standard Doppler is in the location and magnitude of the frequency shift that is identified. For standard Doppler, *the velocity being interrogated is relatively high and the frequency shift produced is large, but the intensity or amplitude of the returning wave is relatively low.* Standard Doppler identifies these signals by using a *high-pass wall filter* to eliminate lower frequency signals, a *high PRF* to avoid aliasing, and a *high gain* to amplify the attenuated signal. For TDI, the velocity of moving myocardium is relatively low and the resultant frequency shift is small, but the amplitude of the returning wave is relatively high. Thus, TDI uses a *low wall filter* to include the signals of interest, a *low PRF* because aliasing is no longer an issue, and *low gain* because there is no need to boost the amplitude of the signal.

5.2 As with flow Doppler, TDI is also angle dependent. Because the most useful and reproducible measure of myocardial motion assessed by TDI is apex-to-base shortening and relaxation, TDI signals are obtained from apical views. The Doppler probe is placed on the septal and lateral LV at the mitral annulus, or at the RV free wall at the tricuspid valve level. A normal TDI signal is comprised of three components: S′, E′, and A′ (Figure 5.1).

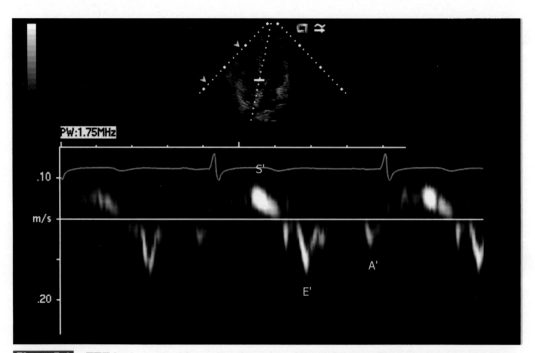

Figure 5.1 TTE in the apical four-chamber view. Normal tissue Doppler imaging at the septal annulus.

S' describes the velocity of base-to-apex shortening that occurs during systole. E' (or Em or Ea) describes the initial reverse motion during the passive-filling phase of early diastole. A' describes the effect of atrial contraction. *Normal values* for E', are ≥ 10 cm/sec for the septum, ≥ 15 cm/sec for the lateral wall, and ≥ 15 cm/sec for the RV free wall. The current utility of TDI centers around its use as a measure of diastolic function (discussed in detail in Sections 10.7–10.9).

5.3   *Myocardial strain* is defined as the change in length of a myocardial segment relative to its initial length. Figure 5.2 shows longitudinal (apex-to-base) systolic shortening, with the resultant change in length of the myocardial segment L_o. Strain is defined as:

$$Strain = \frac{L - L_o}{L_o}$$

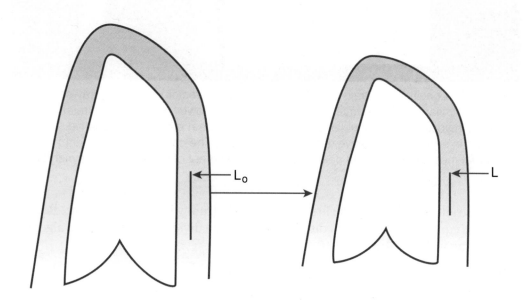

Figure 5.2   Schematic depiction of myocardial strain in which segment L_o shortens to L.

By convention, systolic strain is negative. Units are most commonly reported as percentages (%). Longitudinal strain is measured in the apical view, whereas radial and circumferential strain are measured in the short axis view. A typical longitudinal strain map is shown in Figure 5.3.

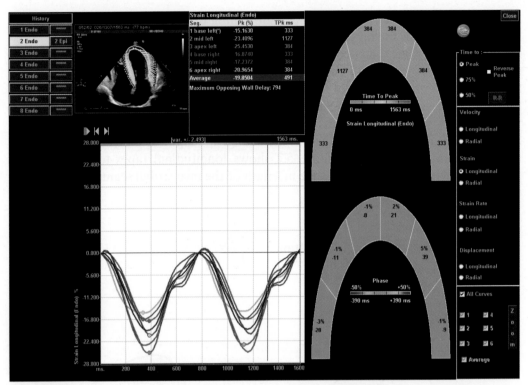

Figure 5.3 Longitudinal strain mapping, using velocity vector imaging, a gray-scale technique similar to speckle tracking. The curves at the lower right show the relative change in myocardial segment length over time. Each beat produces a negative deflection in systole and positive deflection in diastole. The color maps to the right provide segmental measures of time to peak strain for assessment of myocardial dyssynchrony.

5.4 Strain rate is simply the first derivative of strain with respect to time. Because velocity is equal to the change in distance (Δ distance) divided by time, a little algebraic rearranging will give you:

$$\text{strain rate} = \frac{V_1 - V_2}{d}$$

In this equation, d is the distance between the two velocity points. Units are reported as s^{-1}. Strain rate mapped over time is shown in Figure 5.4.

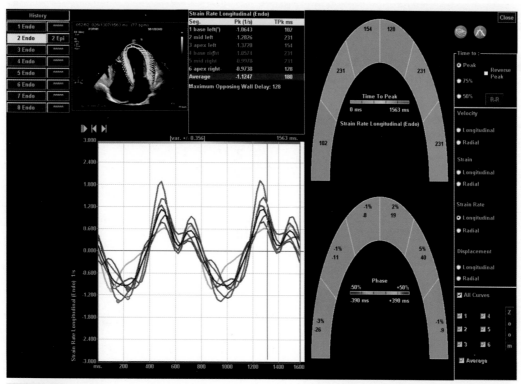

Figure 5.4 Strain rate mapping using velocity vector imaging. The curve produces a single negative deflection in systole and two positive deflections in diastole, akin to E′ and A′.

Systolic strain rate is also negative, and there are two positive diastolic peaks corresponding to passive filling and atrial contraction.

5.5 Thus far, strain and strain rate have provided incremental contributions to clinical echocardiography, but because of their tremendous potential to noninvasively measure small changes in myocardial shortening and relaxation, they hold great promise. The most convincing area where strain has demonstrated this promise is in stress echocardiography, where abnormal strain appears to be the most sensitive and earliest sign of ischemia. You can expect, however, to see much more work emerging in coming years describing myocardial strain and strain rate in a variety of circumstances, including assessment of systolic and diastolic heart failure, longitudinal assessment of LV systolic function in patients receiving chemotherapy and in patients with valvular heart disease, and in further evaluation of response to biventricular pacing.

5.6 *Evaluation of myocardial dyssynchrony*: This technique involves the use of myocardial velocity or strain mapping to look for differences in regional systolic function as a predictor of response to biventricular pacing in advanced heart failure. Multiple criteria for dyssynchrony have been proposed, but initial studies suggesting that dyssynchrony, however measured, can predict biventricular pacing response have not been convincingly reproduced. Current efforts are focused around reevaluating radial strain by speckle tracking.

ADVANCED QUESTION

Q5.4   Choose the correct values for normal diastolic tissue Doppler indices (E′ TDI) from the following table:

	RV free wall (cm)	Septum (cm)	LV free wall (cm)
a.	3	2	5
b.	9	7	5
c.	10	8	3
d.	20	10	15
e.	25	15	10

ANSWER

Q5.4   d: See Section **5.2.**

6

QUANTIFICATION OF CHAMBER VOLUMES, LEFT VENTRICULAR MASS, AND LEFT VENTRICULAR FUNCTION

PRACTICE QUESTIONS

For Question 6.1–6.4, match the quantitative method for calculation of ejection fraction with the appropriate characteristic.

    a.   Teichholz equation

    b.   Area-length equation

    c.   Simpson rule equation

    d.   Penn convention

Q6.1   Will underestimate LV ejection fraction in the setting of an interior wall myocardial infarction.

Q6.2   Best method of estimation of LV ejection fraction when endocardial definition is poor.

Q6.3   Performed exclusively from the apical four chamber view.

Q6.4   Papillary muscles should be excluded when using this method for calculation of LV mass.

ANSWERS: 6.1. a; 6.2. b; 6.3. c; 6.4. b

6.1 To calculate LV mass, the inner (endocardial) volume of the LV is calculated, the outer (epicardial) volume is calculated. The inner volume is subtracted from the outer volume, and the difference is multiplied by the density of blood.

$$\text{LV mass} = 0.8 \times \{1.04[(\text{LVEDD} + \text{ILWT} + \text{SWT})^3 - (\text{LVEDD}^3)]\} + 0.6 \text{ g}$$

In this equation:

- LVEDD = left ventricular end-diastolic dimension

- ILWT = inferolateral wall thickness

- SWT = septal wall thickness

To calculate LV mass using the area-length method, the LV area is planimetered in two planes, multiplied by a constant that assumes the area is an ellipse, and divided by the long axis of the ellipse (Figure 6.1).

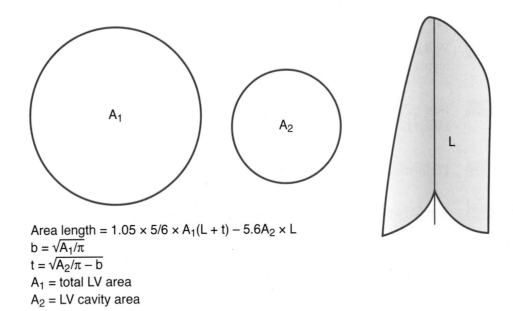

Area length = 1.05 × 5/6 × A₁(L + t) − 5.6A₂ × L
b = √A₁/π
t = √A₂/π − b
A₁ = total LV area
A₂ = LV cavity area

Figure 6.1 Calculation of LV mass using the area length method.

6.2 To calculate LV volume using the short-form area/length method:

$$\text{LV volume} = \frac{0.85(\text{area}^2)}{L}$$

To calculate LV volume using the biplane area/length method:

$$\frac{0.85(A_1)(A_2)}{L}$$

In this equation, A_1 and A_2 are the planimetered areas from the four-chamber and two-chamber views.

6.3   For LA volume, the equation reduces to:

$$\text{LA volume} = \frac{(8)(A_1)(A_2)}{3\pi L}$$

In this equation:

- A_1 = LA area in apical four-chamber view

- A_2 = LA area in apical two-chamber view

- L = shortest atrial length in either the four- or two-chamber view

This equation simplifies to:

$$\text{LA volume} = \frac{0.85(\text{four-chamber area})(\text{two-chamber area})}{\text{shortest atrial length}}$$

LA volume index has prognostic importance in predicting survival after myocardial infarction and the ability to maintain normal sinus rhythm after cardioversion of atrial fibrillation. Increased LA volume index has been shown to be a powerful marker of outcomes in a variety of settings in which LA dimension alone has limited value; it predicts future events in patients hospitalized with heart failure, increased mortality after acute myocardial infarction, increased incidence of atrial fibrillation, increased risk of recurrent atrial fibrillation after cardioversion, increased mortality after acute myocardial infarction, and increased incidence of first ischemic stroke. Even in lone fibrillators, increased LA volume index predicts a higher frequency of adverse cardiac events.

6.4   LV wall thickness is also useful in estimating patterns of hypertrophy using *relative wall thickness*, defined as:

$$\text{Relative wall thickness} = \frac{2(\text{ILWT})}{(\text{LVEDD})}$$

Relative wall thickness can be combined with LV mass index to provide information about pattern of hypertrophy. The chart in Figure 6.2 illustrates that *eccentric hypertrophy* classically produces a pattern of increased LV mass index *with normal relative wall thickness*, whereas concentric hypertrophy produces *increases in both LV mass index and relative wall thickness.*

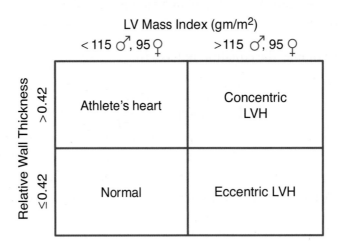

Figure 6.2   Determination of pattern of hypertrophy using relative wall thickness and body mass index. *Source*: Adapted from *J Am Soc Echocardiog* 2005;18:1445.

6.5   *Estimation of LV volumes and ejection fraction*: Three methods of estimating LV volumes and ejection fraction are available: the Teichholtz equation, the area-length equation, and Simpson's rule. They are presented in historic order and increasing frequency of use.

The *Teichholz equation* is an M-mode–derived formula that assumes a spherical shape to the ventricle and produces a volume from standard M-mode measurements:

$$\text{LV end-diastolic volume} = \frac{(\text{LVEDD}^3 \times 7)}{(2.4 + \text{LVEDD})}$$

$$\text{LV end-systolic volume} = \frac{(\text{ESD}^3 \times 7)}{(2.4 + \text{LVESD})}$$

The method assumes that the LV is essentially circular in cross section, a reasonable assumption under most circumstances. Its major limitation is that it also assumes normal wall motion. In a patient with an inferior wall myocardial infarction, for example, the Teichholz equation will produce an LV ejection fraction that is artificially reduced. Conversely, in a patient with an anteroseptal wall myocardial infarction, the equation may produce a normal value for LV ejection fraction when LV function is reduced because the proximal segments when LV dimensions are measured move normally. Given these limitations and the emergence of alternative techniques, the method is largely of historic interest.

6.6   *The area-length method* has been discussed previously in relation to estimation of LV mass. Its major limitation is that it does not account precisely for irregularities in LV shape, but it is the preferred method when the endocardial border is not optimally seen.

6.7   *Simpson's rule or biplane method of discs*: This is the current standard method for quantitation of LV function because it produces highly accurate results and has been automated in most contemporary echocardiographic analysis systems (Figures 6.3a and 6.3b).

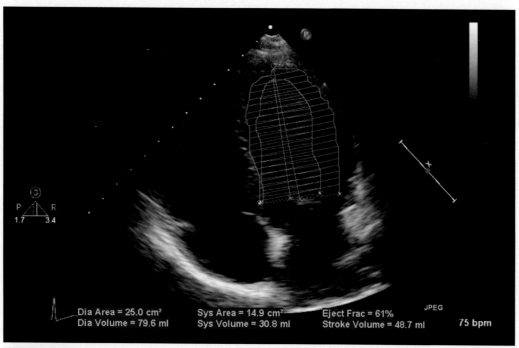

Dia Area = 25.0 cm²   Sys Area = 14.9 cm²   Eject Frac = 61%
Dia Volume = 79.6 ml   Sys Volume = 30.8 ml   Stroke Volume = 48.7 ml   75 bpm

Figure 6.3a   Calculation of LV volumes using the Simpson rule, four-chamber view.

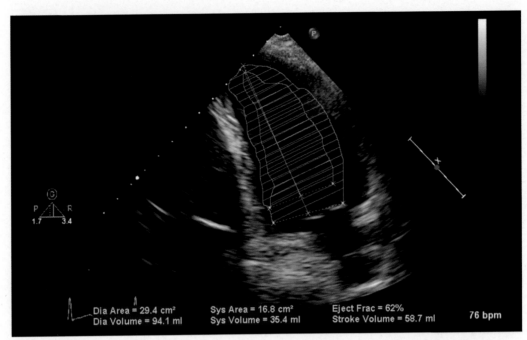

Dia Area = 29.4 cm²
Dia Volume = 94.1 ml

Sys Area = 16.8 cm²
Sys Volume = 35.4 ml

Eject Frac = 62%
Stroke Volume = 58.7 ml

76 bpm

Figure 6.3b   Calculation of LV volumes using the Simpson rule, two-chamber view.

Using automated techniques, this method slices the ventricle into a series of discs, measures the area of each disc, and sums the areas. Mathematically, the formula appears as follows:

$$\text{LV volume} = x\,/\,4 \sum_{i=1} a_i^2 \times \frac{L}{20}$$

Here, a_i equals 20 discs from an apical four- or two-chamber view.

Any ventricular shape, no matter how irregular, will produce a reasonably accurate measure. The method's chief limitation is that it is only as accurate as the endocardial border tracing produced.

Load-Independent Measures of Cardiac Performance

6.8   Any method that mimics or approximates the LV end-systolic pressure-volume relationship can serve as a useful measure of intrinsic LV function. In some arenas, such as timing of aortic or mitral valve replacement or repair in asymptomatic patients, such measures may be critical.

The rate of rise in systolic pressure with time (dP/dt) derived from the spectral–mitral regurgitation gradient. Because the spectral–mitral regurgitation Doppler tracing measures instantaneous pressure, the difference between any two points in systole (the downslope of the tracing) can be used to measure change in pressure, and dividing by the time interval will produce dP/dt. By convention, the time interval is measured between velocities of 1 m/sec and 3 m/sec (the isovolumic phase of contraction), and the numerator is thus fixed at 32 mm Hg: $(4)(3^2) - (4)(1)^2$. Simply divide this number by the measured time interval.

For example, using the findings presented in Figure 6.4:

$$dP / dt = \frac{32 \text{ mm Hg}}{0.025 \text{ sec}} = 1260 \text{ mm Hg} / \text{sec}$$

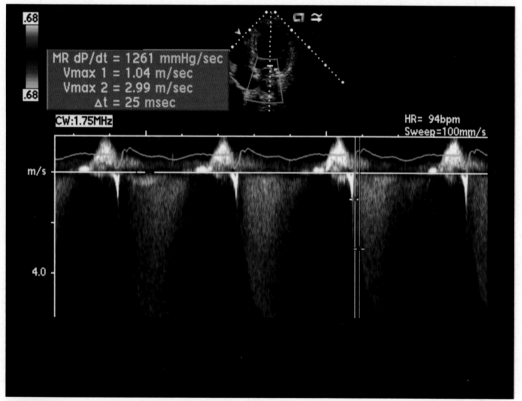

Figure 6.4 Calculation of dP/dt using spectral CW Doppler mitral regurgitation spectral tracing.

Normal dP/dt is 1200 mm Hg/sec or greater.

6.9   *Myocardial performance (or Tei) index* is the ratio of isovolumic contraction time (IVCT) plus isovolumic relaxation time (IVRT) to ejection time (ET) (Figure 6.5).

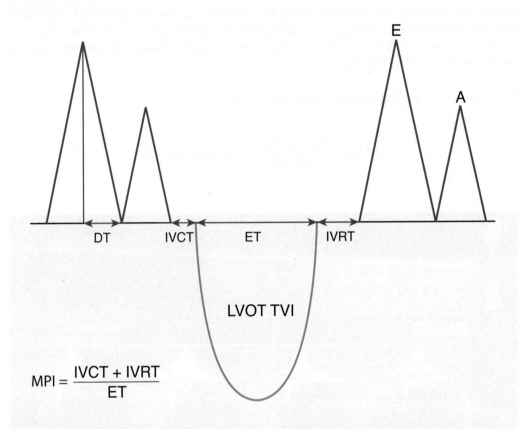

$$MPI = \frac{IVCT + IVRT}{ET}$$

Figure 6.5   Myocardial performance index. Ao, aortic; DT, deceleration time; ET, ejection time; IVCT, isovolumic contraction time; IVRT, isovolumic relaxation time; LVOT, left ventricular outflow tract.

The index, although not reported frequently, has been shown to be a sensitive measure of both decreased systolic function (in which ET and IVCT fall), or diastolic dysfunction (in which IVRT increases). The index is decreased with systolic dysfunction and increased with diastolic dysfunction. The index is independent of heart rate and predicts prognoses in a variety of myopathic disease states. Normal is 0.04 ± 0.005 units.

ADVANCED QUESTIONS

For Questions 6.4–6.7, match the index with the following findings:

    a.   Power/$\sqrt{\text{frequency}}$

    b.   LVOT VTI/aortic valve VTI

    c.   (IVCT + IVRT)/ET

    d.   A value of < 0.25 predicts severe disease.

    e.   This index is calculated from measurements obtained in the four-chamber view.

Q6.4   Mechanical index

Q6.5   Dimensionless index

Q6.6   LA volume index

Q6.7   Myocardial performance (Tei) index

Q6.8   Measurement of dP/dt requires which parameter?

    a.   Mitral regurgitation shown by color Doppler flow

    b.   Mitral regurgitation shown by spectral Doppler flow

    c.   Aortic regurgitation shown by color Doppler flow

    d.   Aortic regurgitation shown by color Doppler flow

    e.   None of the above

Q6.9   Which mathematical relation from the schematic below describes the myocardial performance index?

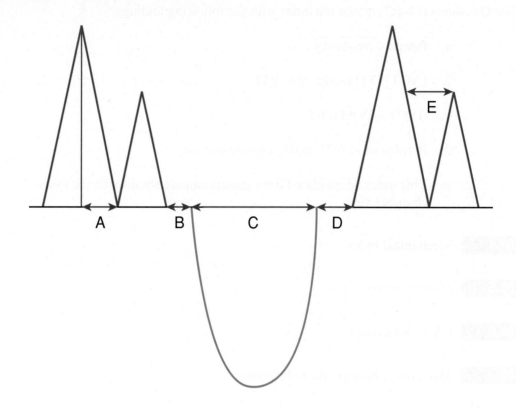

a. $\dfrac{A+B}{C}$

b. $\dfrac{B+C}{D}$

c. $\dfrac{B+D}{C}$

d. $\dfrac{C+D}{B}$

e. $\dfrac{A+D}{C}$

Q6.10   In the prior schematic, which interval measures the IVCT?

    a. A

    b. B

    c. C

    d. D

    e. E

Q6.11   The area-length method for calculation of LV volume and/or mass assumes that the LV has a shape resembling a:

    a. Circle

    b. Sphere

    c. Bullet

    d. Cylinder

    e. Prolate ellipse

Q6.12 Calculate the dP/dt from the information provided in in the image below.

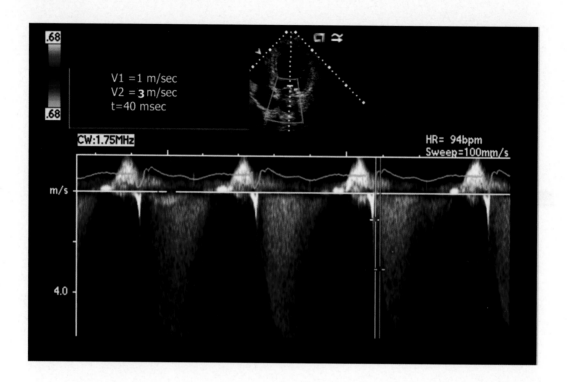

a. 650 mm Hg/sec

b. 800 mm Hg/sec

c. 100 mm Hg/sec

d. 1250 mm Hg/sec

e. 1450 mm Hg/sec

Q6.13   Which combination from the table below best describes a male patient with aortic stenosis and normal systolic function?

LV Mass Index (gm/m^2)

	<115	>115
Relative Wall Thickness >0.42	A	B
Relative Wall Thickness ≤0.42	C	D

a.   A

b.   B

c.   C

d.   D

e.   None of the above

Q6.14   Increased LA volume index is a marker for:

a.   Increased risk for embolic stroke

b.   Increased risk for aortic valve nodal reentrant tachycardia

c.   Increased risk for first myocardial infarction

d.   Increased risk for hospital readmission or death after first admission for heart failure

e.   Increased risk for bleeding after cardiac surgery

ANSWERS

Q6.4   a: For the answers to Questions **6.4–6.7**, see Section **6.9**.

Q6.5   b

Q6.6   e

Q6.7   c

Q6.8   b: See Section **6.8**.

Q6.9   c: The myocardial performance (or Tei) index is described as (IVCT + IVRT)/ET. (Section **6.9**)

Q6.10   b: IVCT is the time from the end of mitral valve closure to aortic valve opening, or the interval between the end of the E wave and the beginning of atrioventricular VTI. (Section **6.9**)

Q6.11   e: Assumption of a prolate ellipse is one of the major limitations of the area-length equation because dilated ventricles are usually more spherical. (Section **6.1**)

Q6.12   b: dP/dt is measured using mitral regurgitation velocities at 1 sec and 3 sec in the example provided and dividing by the time interval between them:

$$\frac{(4)(3\ cm^2) - (4)(1\ cm^2)}{40\ msec}$$

$$= \frac{36\ mm\ Hg - 4\ mm\ Hg}{40\ msec}$$

$$= \frac{32}{0.04\ sec}$$

$$= 800\ mm\ Hg/sec$$

(Section **6.8**)

Q6.13   b: Concentric LV hypertrophy is characterized by increased LV mass with preserved LV cavity size. (Section **6.4**)

Q6.14   d: See Section **6.4**.

7 AORTIC VALVE DISEASE

For Questions 7.1–7.4, match the pattern of LV volume and mass with the appropriate valvular lesion.

    a.   Normal LV volume, normal LV mass

    b.   Increased LV volume, increased LV mass

    c.   Normal LV volume, increased LV mass

    d.   Increased LV volume, normal LV ventricular mass

Q7.1   Aortic stenosis

Q7.2   Aortic regurgitation

Q7.3   Mitral stenosis

Q7.4   Mitral regurgitation

Aortic Stenosis

7.1   Etiologies for aortic stenosis vary with age. In young and middle aged adults, aortic stenosis will most commonly present as the result of congenital anomaly, including bicuspid or, rarely, unicuspid aortic valve. In the elderly, "senile" calcification of a trileaflet valve is the most common cause.

LEARNING DIRECTIVE

See Clip 7.1: A typical example of aortic stenosis. Doming is apparent as the valve bulges in systole. Given the near absence of valvular excursion, the degree of aortic stenosis is likely to be severe.

LEARNING DIRECTIVE

See Clip 7.2: The same valve in short axis view. In contrast to mitral valves, direct aortic valve planimetry is not considered definitive for estimation of aortic valve area because of the difficulty in locating the minimum orifice area. Planimetry by TEE, however, has been validated.

7.2   Although the specific appearance of a bicuspid aortic valve can vary depending upon the closure points, several archetypal findings are commonly seen, including systolic doming, reduced excursion, and eccentric closure in the parasternal long axis view, as in Figure 7.1.

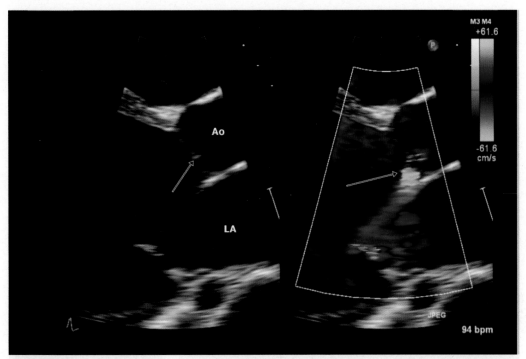

Figure 7.1   TTE parasternal long axis. The eccentric closure point (arrow in left-hand panel) and aortic regurgitation (arrow in right-hand panel) from a bicuspid aortic valve seen in long axis.

LEARNING DIRECTIVE

See Clip 7.6: A bicuspid aortic valve seen in long axis. Note the eccentric closure point.

LEARNING DIRECTIVE

See Clip 7.7: The same valve in short axis. A small raphe of the vestigial third cusp is seen at 11 o'clock.

The diagnosis is most frequently made by visual inspection of the valve in the parasternal short axis view at the level of the aortic valve. The normal triangular opening will be replaced by an oval or "fish mouth" appearance in systole (Figure 7.2a); in diastole, the "peace" sign will be replaced by a single line of closure, often with a vestigial, eccentrically placed raphe representing the absent leaflet. M-mode echocardiography will often demonstrate and eccentric closure point (Figure 7.2b). Aortic stenosis or insufficiency, or both, can be seen in varying degrees.

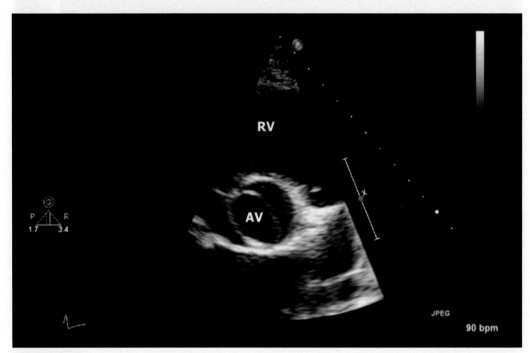

Figure 7.2a   TTE parasternal short axis. A bicuspid aortic valve (AV) in short axis. Note the 10 o'clock to 4 o'clock orientation.

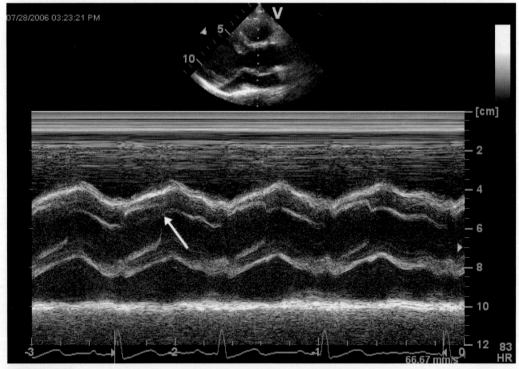

Figure 7.2b   M-mode echocardiography of a bicuspid valve demonstrates an eccentric closure point (arrow).

A unicuspid aortic valve produces an off-center location within the root and an eccentric circular appearance when open (Figure 7.3a). A quadricuspid aortic valve produces an "X" configuration in diastole (Figure 7.3b).

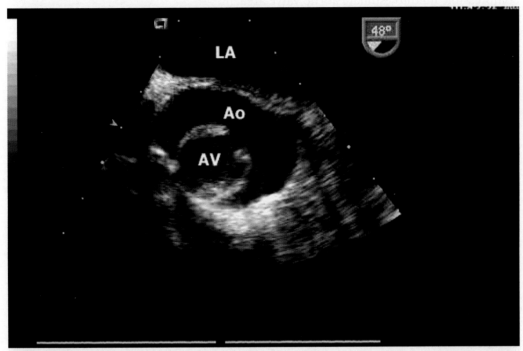

Figure 7.3a   TEE midgastric view at 0°. The off-center circular appearance of a unicuspid aortic valve in systole. Because this is a TEE, the LA lies superior to the aortic root (Ao) and aortic valve (AV).

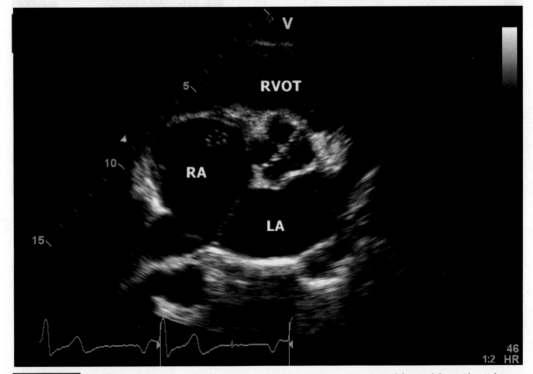

Figure 7.3b   TTE parasternal short axis view demonstrates a quadricuspid aortic valve. RVOT, right ventricular outflow tract.

Calculation of Aortic Valve Area

7.3   The continuity equation uses the principle of conservation of flow of a non-compressible fluid to estimate aortic valve area:

$$A_{AV} \times V_{AV} = A_{LVOT} \times V_{LVOT}$$

In this equation:

- A_{LVOT} = LVOT area

- V_{LVOT} = the VTI or peak velocity across the LVOT (see Figure 4.3)

- A_{AV} = the aortic valve area (what you are solving for)

- VTI_{AV} = the VTI or peak velocity across the aortic valve (Figure 7.4)

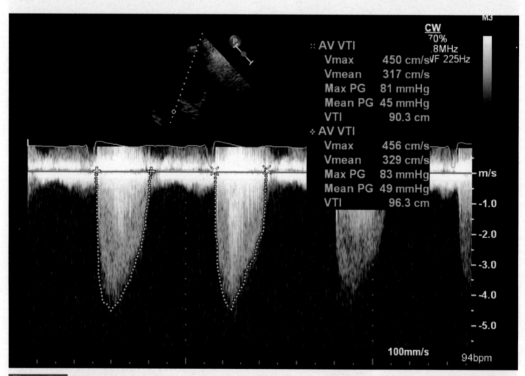

Figure 7.4   The CW Doppler jet across the LVOT in a patient with severe aortic stenosis. The mean and peak velocities and pressure gradients as well as the aortic valve VTI for two beats are shown. Note the slight delay between the onset of the QRS complex and the beginning of the spectral Doppler tracing. The average VTI of the two beats is 93.3 cm.

Solving for aortic valve area, and in the usual detail:

$$\text{aortic valve area} = 0.785 \times (\text{LVOT diameter})^2 \times \frac{\text{VTI}_{\text{LVOT}}}{\text{VTI}_{\text{AV}}}$$

A typical LVOT radius is 1 cm². A typical LVOT peak velocity is 1 m/sec.

Using the data from Chapter 3 and Figure 7.4:

- LVOT diameter = 2.0 cm

- VTI_{LVOT} = 20.7 cm (see Figure 4.3)

you can solve as follows:

$$\text{aortic valve area} = 0.785(2^2)\frac{(20.7)}{(93.3)}$$
$$= 0.7 \text{ cm}^2$$

The continuity equation remains accurate in the presence of any other regurgitant lesion, since flow is still conserved. Either peak gradients or VTI may be used for the flow variable, although VTI will usually produce a slightly smaller valve area. Make sure the value you get makes sense. In general, severe aortic stenosis (aortic valve area ≤ 1.0 cm²) begins at a mean gradient greater than 50 mm Hg, assuming an LVOT diameter of 2 cm² and LVOT velocity of 1 m/sec. If you have a modest gradient and a valve area that is severe, check the variables in the equation to see where the discrepancy is. The LVOT diameter in particular is critical because any error there is squared. Also look to see if the LVOT VTI is really obtained in the proper position. A placement that is too proximal to the valve will artificially increase the degree of aortic stenosis; a placement too distal will have the opposite effect.

7.4   The continuity equation has advantages and disadvantages compared to the Gorlin formula used in the catheterization laboratory. Because CW Doppler measures maximal flow, the gradient measured is the *maximal peak gradient* across the valve, in contrast to the peak aortic to LV gradients obtained in the catheterization laboratory. Consequently, peak gradients obtained in catheterization laboratory tend to be slightly smaller than those obtained using CW Doppler. Mean gradients are similar.

Gradients in the catheterization laboratory are influenced by *pressure recovery*, in which the change in orifice size and the elastic properties of the aorta produce an intrinsic increase in aortic pressure just distal to the stenosis. Doppler flow does not "see" this phenomenon. The net result in the catheterization laboratory is a slightly smaller gradient (usually about 15 mm Hg) and therefore a slightly larger valve area compared to the continuity equation. Factors that increase the magnitude of pressure recovery include the presence of a mechanical prosthesis. Aortic root dilation decreases the effect.

The major advantages of the continuity equation are (1) it does not depend upon accurate measurement of cardiac output because it only looks at relative flow, and (2) for the same reason, it remains accurate in the presence of concomitant aortic regurgitation and mitral regurgitation.

The *dimensionless index* is simply:

$$\text{Aortic valve dimensionless index} = \frac{\text{VTI}_{\text{LVOT}}}{\text{VTI}_{\text{AV}}}$$

The advantage of this quantity is that it eliminates any error from measurement of the LVOT diameter. A dimensionless index less than 0.25 is consistent with severe aortic valve stenosis.

7.5   *Pseudoaortic stenosis*: This entity occurs when stroke volume is very low, leading to reduced LVOT VTI. It results in a continuity equation–derived value for aortic valve area that is low because of reduced flow, and not because true aortic stenosis is present. For example, suppose that a patient produces the following values:

- LVEF = 20%

- $\text{VTI}_{\text{LVOT}} = 15$ cm

- $\text{D}_{\text{LVOT}} = 2$ cm

- Peak atrioventricular gradient = 36 mm Hg, and mean gradient = 18 mm Hg

- $\text{VTI}_{\text{AV}} = 60$ cm

Then:

$$\text{aortic valve area} = \frac{(0.785)(2)^2(15)}{60} = 0.8 \text{ cm}^2$$

Does this patient truly have severe aortic valve stenosis given the modest (6 mm Hg) peak gradient, or is the degree of aortic valve stenosis overestimated because of the patient's reduced stroke volume?

The best technique for distinguishing between these two possibilities is *dobutamine echocardiography*. If the degree of aortic valve stenosis is overestimated, the VTI_{LVOT}

will rise disproportionately to the VTI_{AV} during dobutamine infusion, and the calculated aortic valve area will increase. If the aortic stenosis is correctly estimated, both VTIs will rise in proportion and the aortic valve area will remain unchanged. Dobutamine echocardiography also determines whether myocardial viability is present by demonstrating improvement (or lack thereof) in contractility and/or stroke volume. Examining these two variables—valve area and contractility—together produces three possible outcomes:

1. Pseudoaortic stenosis is present. This condition is straightforward cardiomyopathy, and you treat it as such, regardless of viability.

2. True aortic valve stenosis is present and the myocardium is viable. This patient is referred for aortic valve replacement, with a reasonable expectation that LV systolic function will improve postoperatively.

3. True aortic valve stenosis is present but the myocardium is not viable. In this circumstance, aortic valve replacement may still be recommended as a last resort, but overall results will be less favorable.

Aortic Regurgitation

7.6   Etiologies for aortic regurgitation may be divided between those disease states in which abnormalities within the valve itself are the cause of the insufficiency and those disease states in which aortic regurgitation is the result of proximal abnormalities within the aortic root or downstream abnormalities within the ascending aorta. The former causes include congenital anomalies such as bicuspid aortic valve disease, degenerative aortic valve disease, rheumatic heart disease, rheumatologic diseases (including rheumatoid arthritis and systemic lupus erythematosus), and endocarditis. The latter etiologies include Marfan syndrome, aortic aneurysm, aortic dissection, and ankylosing spondylitis.

7.7   Echocardiographic signs of severe aortic regurgitation are multiple and depend upon both the degree of severity of regurgitation and the rate of onset.

1. *Early diastolic aortic valve opening (when severe aortic regurgitation is acute)*: seen because LV diastolic pressure rises above aortic diastolic pressure

2. *Premature mitral valve closure (again, when severe aortic regurgitation is acute)*: also seen because LV diastolic pressure rises above aortic diastolic pressure; best recognized by M-mode, in which the normal M and W shape of the mitral valve contracts to a diamond

See Clip 7.11: Mitral valve M-mode in the setting of severe acute aortic regurgitation. The diamond-shaped pattern demonstrates early mitral valve closure, a classic sign of acutely increased diastolic pressure caused by acute aortic regurgitation.

1. Color Doppler aortic regurgitation width/LVOT diameter > 50% (Figure 7.5)

See Clip 7.13: Severe aortic insufficiency by color Doppler flow.

2. Pressure half-time < 200 msec: a relatively nonspecific sign because it is load sensitive (Figure 7.6)

3. Aortic regurgitation jet vena contracta width > 0.6 cm

4. Effective regurgitant orifice (ERO) (by proximal isovelocity surface area [PISA]) > 0.3 cm^2

5. Aortic regurgitant volume > 60 ml

6. Aortic regurgitant fraction ≥ 55%

7. LV end-diastolic dimension > 7.5 cm

8. LV end-systolic dimension > 5.5 cm

9. *Diastolic flow reversal in the aorta* (Figure 7.7)

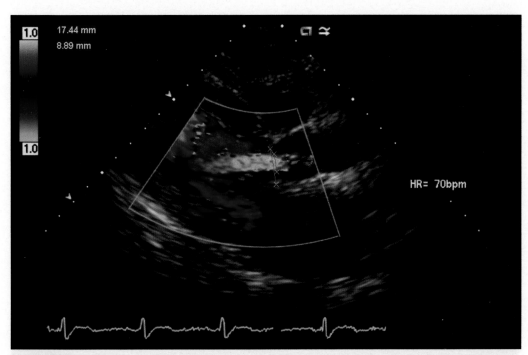

Figure 7.5   TTE parasternal long axis. Estimation of the severity of aortic regurgitation by estimating the ratio of aortic regurgitation jet width to the LVOT diameter. In this patient, the ratio is 8.9/17.4 = 50%, fulfilling the criteria for severe aortic regurgitation.

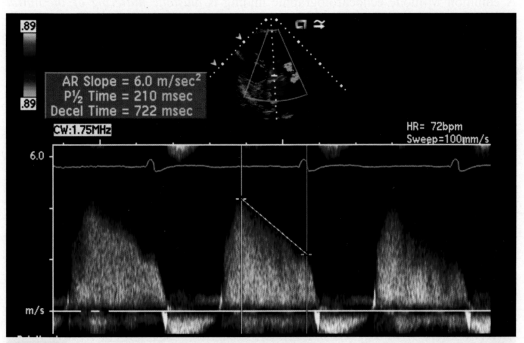

Figure 7.6   The spectral Doppler jet of severe aortic regurgitation. The short pressure half-time (~200 msec) is consistent with the diagnosis.

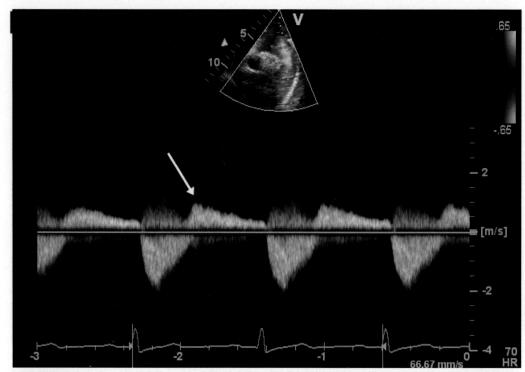

Figure 7.7 Spectral Doppler of flow in the descending aorta demonstrates diastolic flow reversal (arrow).

A common M-mode echocardiographic finding is *diastolic fluttering of the mitral valve*, caused by the flow of the regurgitant jet against the anterior mitral valve leaflet (Figure 7.8).

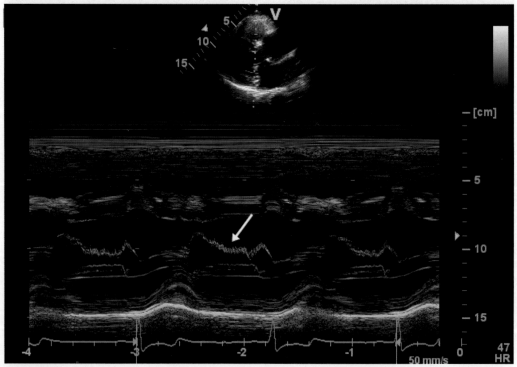

Figure 7.8 M-mode echocardiography demonstrates diastolic fluttering of the anterior mitral valve leaflet in the setting of aortic regurgitation (arrow).

7.8   Quantitative methods for calculating aortic regurgitation include estimation of *ERO* by subtracting the mitral valve inflow from the aortic valve outflow.

First, calculate the aortic stroke volume (SV_{AV}):

$$(0.785)(\text{LVOT diameter})^2(\text{VTI}_{LVOT})$$

Next, calculate mitral valve (MV) stroke volume (SV_{MV}):

$$(0.785)(\text{MV annulus diameter})^2(\text{VTI}_{MV})$$

Subtract the two:

$$\text{regurgitant volume}_{AV} = SV_{AV} - SV_{MV}$$

$$\text{regurgitant fraction}_{AV} = \frac{\text{regurgitant volume}_{AV}}{SV_{AV}}$$

And since:

$$\text{flow} \times \text{area} = \text{volume}$$

we can solve ERO as:

$$\text{ERO} = \frac{\text{atrioventricular regurgitant volume}_{AV}}{\text{VTI}_{AV}}$$

The same calculation works for estimation of ERO in mitral regurgitation, as we will see in the next chapter; however, in that case, aortic valve stroke volume is subtracted from mitral valve stroke volume. This method does not work *if the other valve is also regurgitant*, since its true stroke volume cannot be calculated in that circumstance.

(Calculation of ERO in the setting of a regurgitant lesion using PISA is explained in detail in Section 8.15).

7.9   The pattern of LV hypertrophy associated with aortic regurgitation differs distinctly from aortic stenosis. In aortic stenosis, the pressure load produces sarcomeres laid down in parallel, and the hypertrophy is *concentric* with a normal cavity size. In aortic regurgitation, sarcomeres are laid down in series, and the hypertrophy is *eccentric* with an ever-increasing end-diastolic volume.

ADVANCED QUESTIONS

Use the following data for Questions 7.5–7.7:

$$VTI_{LVOT} = 40 \text{ cm}$$

$$D_{LVOT} = 1.8 \text{ cm}$$

$$VTI_{AV} = 96 \text{ cm}$$

$$VTI_{MV} = 28 \text{ cm}$$

$$Diameter_{MV} = 2 \text{ cm}$$

Q7.5   The aortic valve regurgitant stroke volume is:

a.   15 ml

b.   25 ml

c.   35 ml

d.   45 ml

e.   It cannot be calculated in the absence of mitral regurgitation.

Q7.6   The aortic regurgitant fraction is:

a.   15%

b.   35%

c.   45%

d.   It cannot be calculated in the absence of mitral regurgitation.

Q7.7   The aortic valve ERO is:

a.   0.15 cm^2

b.   0.25 cm^2

c.   0.35 cm^2

d.   0.45 cm^2

e.   It cannot be calculated in the absence of mitral regurgitation

Q7.8   Consider the following values in a patient referred for a dobutamine echocardiogram for evaluation of pseudoaortic stenosis ("low-output" aortic stenosis):

	Rest	Dobutamine 10 ug/kg/min
VTI_{LVOT}	30 cm	35 cm
VTI_{AV}	120 cm	140 cm
LVEF	20%	20%

What would you recommend?

   a.   Cardiac catheterization

   b.   Aortic valve replacement with expectation of an excellent outcome

   c.   No recommendation because data are incomplete

   d.   Aortic valve replacement as a last resort because outcome is less favorable

   e.   TEE for direct aortic valve planimetered

Q7.9   The most likely finding to produce pressure recovery is:

   a.   Subaortic stenosis

   b.   Bicuspid valve

   c.   Mechanical prosthesis

   d.   Apical hypertrophic cardiomyopathy

   e.   Aortic insufficiency

Q7.10   In distinguishing the spectral Doppler signal of mitral regurgitation from aortic stenosis, the most useful characteristic of the jet is:

   a.   Width

   b.   Velocity

   c.   Density

   d.   Location

   e.   Presence of aliasing

Q7.11   The two M-mode echocardiograms shown in Figure Q7.11 were obtained six months apart in the same patient. What clinical condition is demonstrated by the M-mode tracing in part b?

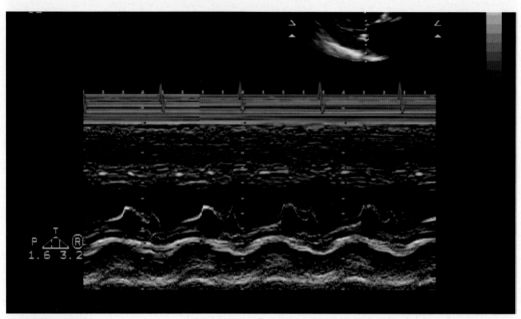

Figure Q7.11a

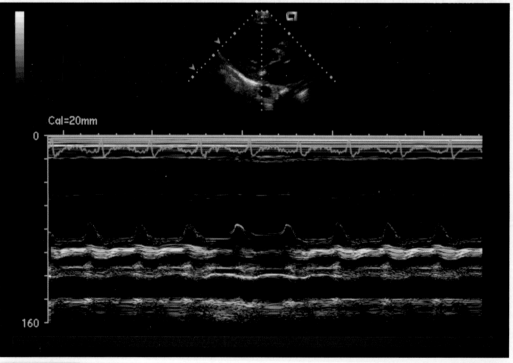

Figure Q7.11b

a. Acute mitral regurgitation

b. Acute aortic regurgitation

c. Acute tricuspid regurgitation

d. Acute pulmonic regurgitation

e. Acute myocardial infarction

Q7.12   In a patient with aortic stenosis, the valve area obtained from the Gorlin formula in the catheterization laboratory is higher than the valve area obtained by echocardiography using the continuity equation. This discrepancy is explained by:

a. Mitral regurgitation

b. Aortic regurgitation

c. Diastolic dysfunction

d. Hypertension

e. Pressure recovery

Q7.13   Calculate the aortic valve area from the following data:

$$D_{LVOT} = 2.2 \text{ cm}$$

$$VTI_{LVOT} = 20 \text{ cm}$$

$$VTI_{LVOT} / VTI_{AV} = 0.2$$

$$VTI_{AV} = 100 \text{ cm}$$

Moderate aortic regurgitation is present.

a. Aortic valve area $= 1.1 \text{ cm}^2$

b. Aortic valve area $= 1.0 \text{ cm}^2$

c. Aortic valve area $= 0.8 \text{ cm}^2$

d. Aortic valve area cannot be calculated because sufficient data are not provided.

e. Aortic valve area cannot be calculated because of the presence of aortic regurgitation.

Q7.14 The pressure gradient measured across the aortic valve during calculation of the continuity equation corresponds to which measured gradient in the catheterization laboratory?

    a. Mean gradient

    b. Peak instantaneous gradient

    c. Peak-to-peak gradient

    d. None of the above

    e. All of the above

Q7.15 Calculating the aortic valve area using the continuity equation requires measurement of the VTI at the level of the LVOT and at the level of the aortic valve. When recording the VTI of LVOT, positioning the sample volume too close to the aortic valve will result in an aortic valve area that:

    a. Underestimates aortic valve area

    b. Overestimates aortic valve area

    c. Underestimates aortic valve mean gradient

    d. Underestimates aortic valve peak gradient

    e. Has no effect on calculation of aortic valve area or aortic valve gradient

ANSWERS

Q7.5   a

Regurgitant stroke volume = atrioventricular outflow − mitral valve inflow

$$= (0.785)(D_{LVOT})^2(TV_{LVOT}) - (0.785)(D_{MV})^2(VTI_{MV})$$

$$= (0.785)(1.8)^2(40) - (0.785)(2)^2(28)$$

$$= 102 \text{ ml} - 88 \text{ ml}$$

$$= 14 \text{ ml}$$

(Section **7.8**)

Q7.6   a

$$\text{Regurgitant fraction} = \frac{\text{regurgitant volume}}{\text{stroke volume}}$$

$$= \frac{14 \text{ ml}}{102 \text{ ml}}$$

$$= 15\%$$

(Section **7.8**)

Q7.7   a

$$\text{ERO} = \frac{\text{regurgitant volume}}{\text{regurgitant VTI}}$$

$$= \frac{14 \text{ cm}^3}{96 \text{ cm}}$$

$$= 0.15 \text{ cm}^2$$

(Section **7.8**)

Q7.8   d: Note that the LVOT diameter is not provided. You do not need it to calculate the relative stroke volume at rest and with low-dose dobutamine because it does not change. At rest:

$$\frac{\text{VTI}_{\text{LVOT}}}{\text{VTI}_{\text{AV}}} = \frac{30}{120} = 0.25$$

With dobutamine:

$$\frac{\text{VTI}_{\text{LVOT}}}{\text{VTI}_{\text{AV}}} = \frac{35}{140} = 0.25$$

Increased LVOT VTI with dobutamine:

$$\frac{35-30}{30} = 15\%$$

These values tell you that true aortic stenosis is present but that myocardial viability is quite limited. Aortic valve replacement may still be attempted but will produce a less favorable outcome. (Section **7.5**)

Q7.9   c: Pressure recovery is accentuated in the presence of a mechanical prosthesis. (Section **7.4**)

Q7.10   a: The mitral regurgitation jet is always wider than the aortic stenosis jet in the same patient because the mitral regurgitation jet commences immediately after the onset of systole. (Section **8.11**)

Q7.11   b: Premature mitral valve closure is a hallmark of acute aortic regurgitation, as the sudden rise in LV diastolic pressure forces the mitral valve to close early. (Section **7.7**)

Q7.12   e: Pressure recovery reduces the aortic valve gradient and therefore produces a slightly larger valve area. (Section **7.4**)

Q7.13   c

$$\text{aortic valve area} = (0.785)(\text{D}_{\text{LVOT}})^2 \frac{(\text{VTI}_{\text{LVOT}})}{\text{VTI}_{\text{AV}}}$$

$$= (0.785)(2.2\ \text{cm}^2)(0.2)$$

$$= 0.76\ \text{cm}^2$$

Obviously, several bits of extra or misleading data were included. (Section **7.3**)

Q7.14   b: See Section **7.4**.

Q7.15   b: If the LVOT gradient is measured too close to the aortic valve (so that part of the aortic stenosis gradient is actually measured), the TV_{LVOT}:VTI_{AV} ratio will be larger than it should be, and the aortic valve area will appear larger than it actually is. (Section **7.3**)

PRACTICE QUESTIONS

Q8.1 In patients with rheumatic mitral stenosis, a scoring system composed of four components is used to determine the suitability of the valve for mitral valvuloplasty. The severity of each component is assessed on a 1–4 scale. Which of the following correctly lists those four components?

a. Mitral leaflet mobility, mitral valve area, mitral calcification, subvalvular involvement

b. Mitral leaflet mobility, mitral leaflet thickening, mitral valve calcification, severity of mitral regurgitation

c. Mitral leaflet mobility, mitral leaflet thickening, severity of mitral regurgitation, subvalvular involvement

d. Mitral leaflet mobility, mitral leaflet thickening, mitral calcification, subvalvular involvement

e. Mitral leaflet mobility, mitral leaflet thickening, mitral annular calcification, mitral valve calcification

Q8.2 Which of the following is a reliable M-mode sign of rheumatic deformity?

a. Decreased E-point septal separation

b. Increased E-point septal separation

c. Diastolic anterior motion of the posterior mitral valve leaflet

d. Aortic valve notching

e. Diastolic fluttering of the anterior mitral leaflet

Q8.3   Which TTE view can produce a false-positive finding of mitral valve prolapse?

   a.   Parasternal long axis

   b.   Parasternal short axis

   c.   Apical three-chamber

   d.   Apical four-chamber

   e.   Subcostal

Rheumatic Mitral Valve Disease and Mitral Stenosis

8.1   The pathology of rheumatic mitral valve disease is well reflected by its echocardiographic characteristics. The disease process begins as fusion of the commisures at the leaflets' tips. Over time, the rheumatic process may spread toward the base of the leaflets and extend down into the subchordal apparatus to produce the characteristic "hockey stick" deformity or doming appearance of the anterior leaflet and poor leaflet mobility (Figure 8.1a). Rheumatic mitral regurgitation is more common than hemodynamically significant mitral stenosis. The M-mode hallmark of rheumatic mitral stenosis is *diastolic anterior motion of the posterior leaflet* as the posterior leaflet tip is pulled anteriorly by its fusion to the anterior leaflet (Figure 8.1b). The M-mode tracing of the mitral valve loses its characteristic "M and W" shape and looks more like a parallelogram.

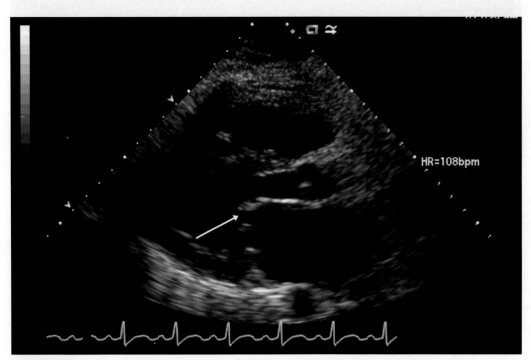

Figure 8.1a   TTE parasternal long axis view of rheumatic deformity of the mitral valve leaflets. Note the diastolic doming of the anterior valve leaflet (arrow).

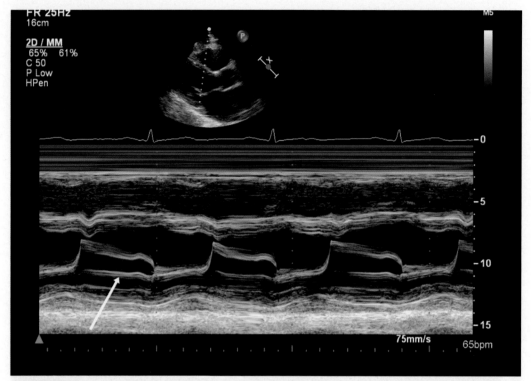

Figure 8.1b TTE parasternal long axis M-mode tracing of rheumatic mitral stenosis. Note anterior motion of the posterior mitral leaflet (arrow).

LEARNING DIRECTIVE

See Clip 8.6: 2D echocardiogram of the same valve shown in Clip 8.5. There is leaflet thickening, mild doming, and mildly decreased leaflet opening.

Less common forms of mitral stenosis include congenital mitral stenosis seen in the young and middle-aged, and senile functional calcific mitral stenosis in which severe mitral annular calcification ultimately intrudes upon the valve orifice, seen in the elderly. Congenital mitral stenosis may occur either as the result of valvular hypoplasia or as a function of abnormalities of the valvular substructure such as chordal shortening or parachute mitral valve.

8.2   Calculation of mitral valve area can be accomplished using several techniques, including:

1. Direct 2D planimetry

2. Pressure half-time method

3. PISA with angle correction

4. Continuity equation equating mitral inflow with aortic outflow

8.3   The *pressure half-time method* relates the rate of pressure decline across the mitral valve to the area of the orifice. The pressure half-time is determined by measuring the time required for the peak pressure to drop in half. To calculate the velocity at which that pressure drop occurs, it is useful to recall that just as pressure across an orifice increases as a function of the square of the velocity of flow across the orifice, pressure decreases as a function *of the square root of the velocity across the orifice.*

If $P_{max} = 4V_{max}{}^2$, then $V_{max}{}^2 = P_{max}/4$.

If $V_{1/2}$ = the velocity at which the pressure has dropped in half, then:

$$V_{1/2}^2 = \tfrac{1}{2}(P_{max}/4)$$

$$V_{1/2}^2 = \tfrac{1}{2}(4V_{max}^2/4)$$

$$V_{1/2}^2 = \tfrac{1}{2}V_{max}^2$$

$$V_{1/2} = V_{max}/\sqrt{2}$$

or:

$$V_{1/2} = \frac{V_{max}}{1.41}, \text{ or } 0.71V_{max}$$

The pressure half-time is determined by measuring the time interval between V_{max} and $V_{1/2}$ (Figure 8.1c).

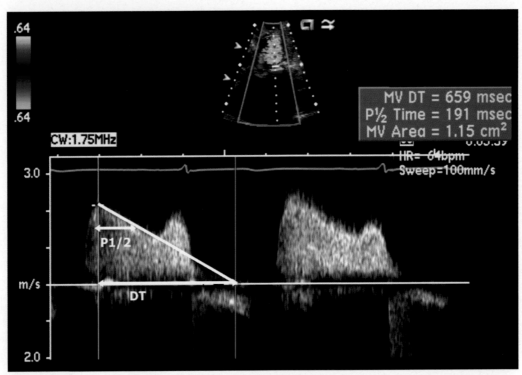

Figure 8.1c The pressure halftime ($P_{\frac{1}{2}}$) is determined by measuring the time interval required for the peak pressure to drop in half. DT, deceleration time.

Mitral valve area is estimated by dividing an empiric constant, 220, by the pressure half-time:

$$\text{mitral valve area} = \frac{220}{\text{pressure half-time}}$$

The constant, derived by Liv Hatle, was based upon a series of observations in patients with rheumatic mitral stenosis. This last detail is important because the Hatle constant does not hold for mitral stenosis produced by other etiologies.

8.4 The geometry of a right triangle determines that the mitral deceleration time (the time from initial mitral inflow velocity to equilibration between LV and LA) is related to both the pressure half-time and the mitral valve area (Figure 8.2).

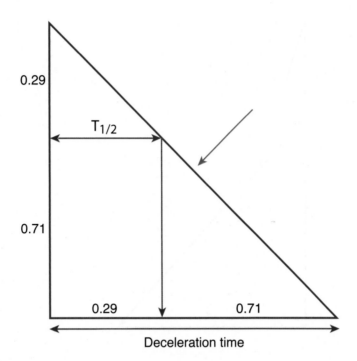

Figure 8.2   The geometric relationship between the pressure half-time and the deceleration time (arrow).

This relationship allows the pressure half-time and mitral valve area to be calculated directly from the deceleration time alone:

$$\text{pressure half-time} = 0.29 \times \text{deceleration time}$$

and:

$$\text{mitral valve area} = \frac{750}{\text{deceleration time}}$$

If the slope of the pressure decline is biphasic, the second, shallower slope should be used to estimate the deceleration time (Figure 8.3).

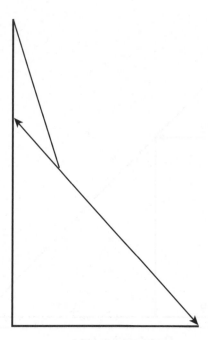

Figure 8.3   Proper estimation using the shallower second slope of the mitral valve inflow tracing when it is biphasic.

The pressure half-time method critically assumes that diastolic function is normal. In a patient with diastolic dysfunction or decreased compliance, the method underestimates the degree of mitral stenosis (overestimates the mitral valve area) because the rate at which diastolic pressure rises artificially shortens the pressure half-time. Severe aortic regurgitation has the same effect by the same mechanism.

8.5   The *PISA method* uses the continuity equation (see section 8.15 for a detailed explanation), except in this instance, an angle correction must be added to account for the fact that the surface area of the hemisphere of flow is reduced by the angle between the two stenotic valve leaflets. The angle is estimated or measured directly from the stenotic mitral valve leaflets (Figure 8.4).

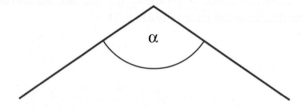

Figure 8.4   Using PISA to calculate mitral valve area in mitral stenosis.

The PISA equation modifies to:

$$ERO = \frac{(6.28)(\text{PISA radius})(\text{aliasing velocity}) \times (a)}{(\text{peak mitral valve inflow gradient})(180°)}$$

8.6   In the *continuity equation method* mitral valve (MV) inflow is equal to LVOT valve outflow. It is calculated as follows:

$$(MVA)(VTI_{MV}) = (A_{LVOT})(VTI_{LVOT})$$

$$MVA = \frac{(0.785)(D_{LVOT})^2(VTI_{LVOT})}{VTI_{MV}}$$

8.7   The *mitral valvuloplasty scoring system* is used for determining the suitability of a stenotic mitral valve for percutaneous valvuloplasty. It has four components, each worth 4 points with a total scoring range of 4–16. The score for each component is determined as follows: 1 = normal, 2 = mildly abnormal, 3 = moderately abnormal, and 4 = severely abnormal. The components are:

a.   Leaflet thickening

b.   Leaflet mobility

c.   Leaflet calcification

d.   Subvalvular thickening

The severity of mitral regurgitation is *not* one of the criteria, although patients with at least moderate mitral regurgitation are generally not good candidates for percutaneous balloon mitral valvuloplasty. A score of 8 or less is usually favorable for valvuloplasty in the absence of moderate or greater mitral regurgitation.

Mitral Regurgitation

8.8   The echocardiographic appearance of a regurgitant mitral valve often explains the mechanism of regurgitation. Most common etiologies for mitral regurgitation include (in descending order of frequency in the present era):

a.   Ischemic heart disease/acute myocardial infarction

b.   Myxomatous degeneration/mitral valve prolapse

  c. Endocarditis

  d. Functional mitral regurgitation from LV dilatation or cardiomyopathy

  e. Rheumatic mitral valve disease

  f. Congenital anomalies such as parachute mitral valve or cleft mitral leaflet

8.9 When mitral regurgitation is due to differential malfunction or malcoaptation of one leaflet, such as posterior leaflet tethering from an inferior wall myocardial infarction or flail leaflet as the result of a ruptured chordae tendinea, the regurgitant jet will flow in the direction *opposite* to the affected leaflet (Figure 8.5).

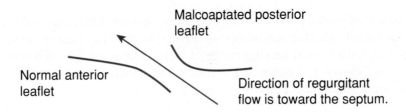

Malcoaptated posterior leaflet

Normal anterior leaflet

Direction of regurgitant flow is toward the septum.

Figure 8.5 The direction of regurgitant flow moves away from the affected leaflet.

By contrast, mitral regurgitation as the result of LV dilatation in the setting of cardiomyopathy will usually produce a central jet.

8.10 The incidence of *mitral valve prolapse* has declined sharply from earliest estimates, as the fidelity of TTE has combined with more stringent criteria to produce a more accurate measure. Current criteria define mitral valve prolapse as bowing of 2 mm or greater in either mitral valve leaflet below the line created in systole by the normally closed valve (Figure 8.6).

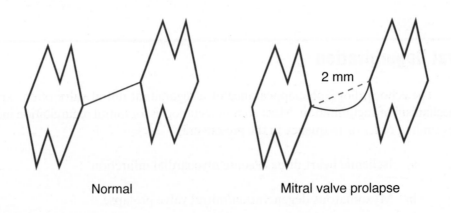

Normal

2 mm

Mitral valve prolapse

Figure 8.6 Schematic of the M-mode appearance and criteria for mitral valve prolapse.

See Clip 8.2b: Holosystolic mitral valve prolapse by 2D echocardiogram.

LEARNING DIRECTIVE

Whether by 2D or M-mode, the measurement is made in the parasternal long axis view because the saddle shape of the mitral valve in the closed position can produce a false-positive result from the apical view. Although the finding is not universally accepted, several studies have reported an association between mitral valve prolapse and increased risk of sudden cardiac death.

8.11   While the mitral regurgitant volume varies widely across the spectrum of disease severity, the pressure gradient will always be the difference between systolic blood pressure and LA pressure, and the onset of the mitral regurgitation jet will occur simultaneously with the initiation of the QRS complex. By contrast, the onset of an aortic stenosis jet begins after the R wave because of the time required for LV pressure to increase and exceed the aortic pressure gradient.

8.12   *Definite criteria for severe mitral regurgitation*:

1. Color Doppler mitral regurgitation $\dfrac{\text{jet area}}{\text{LA area}} > 40\%$ (the weakest criterion)

2. Vena contract > 0.7 mm

3. ERO measured by PISA > 0.4 cm^2

4. Mitral regurgitant volume > 60 ml

5. Regurgitant fraction > 55%

6. Pulmonary vein flow reversal during ventricular systole

8.13   *Ancillary criteria* (supportive findings):

1. LA enlargement (LA dimension > 55 mm)

2. Coanda effect for eccentric jets

3. Dense CW Doppler signal

4. Restrictive mitral valve inflow pattern (deceleration time < 140 msec) as the result of elevated LA pressure

5. For prosthetic mitral regurgitation, high peak mitral inflow with normal deceleration time

6. Tenting area greater than 6 cm^2 for functional mitral regurgitation

Methods for Quantification of Mitral Regurgitation

8.14 *The ratio of mitral regurgitation color jet area to LA area*: Also referred to as the method of Singh (Figure 8.7) from the original reference. This is the most common "eyeball" method that we use on a daily basis, but it is the least accurate. The cutoffs are:

- Trivial mitral regurgitation < 10%

- Mild mitral regurgitation 10–20%

- Moderate mitral regurgitation 20–40%

- Severe mitral regurgitation > 40%

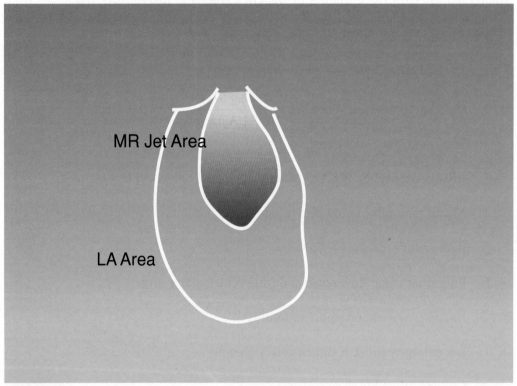

Figure 8.7 Estimation of mitral valve area using the ratio of mitral regurgitation jet area to LA area.

This method assumes the jet is central, or at least not markedly eccentric. Eccentric jets measured by this method in particular will be underestimated because they will tend to obey the Coanda effect (Figure 8.8), in which a volume of flow intersecting a curved surface (such as the posterior wall of the LA) will spread along the contour of that surface, artificially reducing its area.

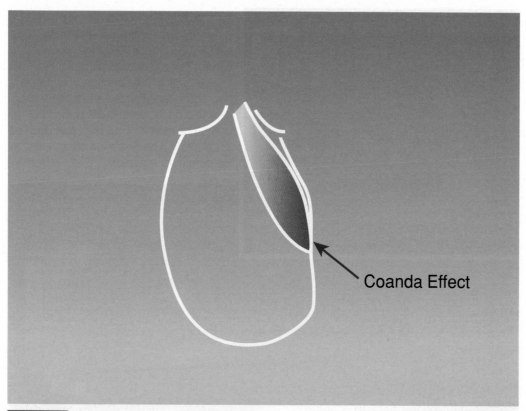

Figure 8.8   Schematic of the Coanda effect.

LEARNING DIRECTIVE

See Clip 8.25: Severe mitral regurgitation is artificially reduced in area by the left atrial wall boundary, an example of the Coanda effect.

8.15   *Mitral regurgitation by PISA*: If the technical quality is good, this is a highly accurate quantitative method. The key to understanding PISA is to remember that the atrioventricular pressure gradient across the regurgitant mitral orifice is much greater than the pressure gradient across the LVOT. Consequently the regurgitant volume flows *at a higher velocity* across the regurgitant mitral valve than the normal stroke volume flows out the LVOT. Because the regurgitant volume flows at a high velocity, it will alias when interrogated at a low enough Nyquist limit. The differential in aliasing velocity between mitral regurgitation and aortic outflow will produce a detectable boundary between the regurgitant flow and the normal aortic outflow. You find that boundary by turning down the PRF or Nyquist limit of the color map to < 40 cm/sec so that aliasing of the mitral regurgitation flow volume occurs, and a semicircle of color consolidates above the valve on the ventricular side (Figure 8.9).

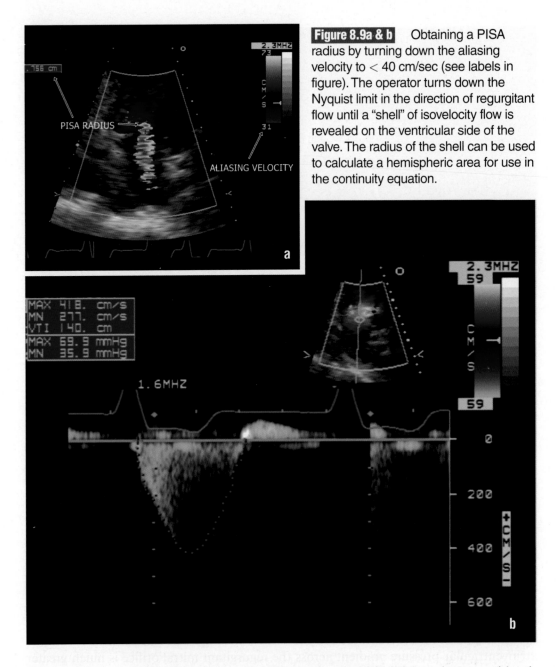

Figure 8.9a & b Obtaining a PISA radius by turning down the aliasing velocity to < 40 cm/sec (see labels in figure). The operator turns down the Nyquist limit in the direction of regurgitant flow until a "shell" of isovelocity flow is revealed on the ventricular side of the valve. The radius of the shell can be used to calculate a hemispheric area for use in the continuity equation.

The semicircle is defined by the fact that all the blood within it is moving at an identical velocity, or isovelocity. This isovelocity "shell" roughly has the shape of a hemisphere, and its surface area is thus calculated as $2\pi r^2$ (or $6.28r^2$), where the radius is the distance from the vena contracta to the outer edge of the shell. Now you have all the variables you need to calculate the ERO using the continuity equation.

Flow proximal to the regurgitant orifice is calculated as:

$$(6.28)(\text{isovelocity radius}^2)(\text{aliasing velocity})$$

You read these variables directly off the screen as shown in Figure 8.9a.

The velocity of the regurgitant jet is measured from the spectral CW Doppler tracing of the mitral regurgitation jet (Figure 8.9b).

$$\text{regurgitant volume} = (\text{ERO})(\text{regurgitant jet VTI})$$

Using the data from Figures 8.9a and 8.9b:

$$\text{ERO} = \frac{(6.28)(r^2)(\text{aliasing radius})}{\text{regurgitant jet peak velocity}}$$

$$= \frac{(6.28)(0.756 \text{ cm}^2)(31 \text{ cm/sec})}{418 \text{ cm/sec}}$$

$$= 0.26 \text{ cm}^2$$

regurgitant volume is calculated as:

$$(\text{ERO})(\text{regurgitant jet VTI}) = (0.26 \text{ cm}^2)(140 \text{ cm}) = 36 \text{ cc}$$

The threshold for severe mitral regurgitation is an ERO > 0.40 cm^2, which has been reported to be predictive of increased mortality, and which represents a commonly used cutoff for mitral valve repair or replacement.

8.16 *Estimation of mitral regurgitation by subtraction of systolic LVOT outflow from diastolic mitral valve inflow*: First, calculate aortic stroke volume as the flow through the LVOT:

$$(0.785)(D_{LVOT})^2(VTI_{LVOT})$$

Then calculate mitral valve inflow stroke volume:

$$(0.785)(D_{MV})^2(VTI_{MV})$$

Then subtract the two:

$$MV_{\text{regurgitant volume}} = SV_{MV} - SV_{LVOT}$$

$$MV_{\text{regurgitant fraction}} = \frac{MV_{\text{regurgitant volume}}}{SV_{MV}}$$

And because volume = flow × area:

$$\text{ERO} = \frac{MV_{\text{regurgitant volume}}}{VTI_{MV}}$$

The same calculation works for estimation of isolated aortic regurgitation, except in that case, LVOT stroke volume is subtracted from mitral valve stroke volume. Note that this method does not work *if the aortic and mitral valves are both regurgitant* because its true stroke volume cannot be calculated.

8.17 *Diastolic mitral regurgitation* (Figure 8.10) occurs when the normal diastolic gradient across the mitral valve gradient is delayed or reversed, either as the result of abnormal timing of atrial relaxation, as in atrioventricular block, or as a consequence of an abnormal rate of decline in LV pressure, as in acute severe aortic regurgitation or constrictive pericarditis.

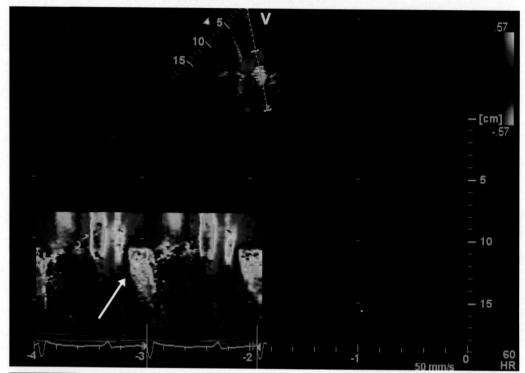

Figure 8.10 Color Doppler flow demonstrating diastolic mitral regurgitation in a patient with complete heart block.

LEARNING DIRECTIVE

See Clip 8.29: Diastolic mitral regurgitation in a patient with high degree atrioventricular block.

ADVANCED QUESTIONS

Q8.4 Which of the following statements regarding the pressure half-time method for estimation of mitral stenosis is true?

a. The method overestimates mitral valve area if LV compliance is decreased.

b. Mitral valve area cannot be estimated from the deceleration time alone.

c. The method is accurate in the presence of aortic regurgitation.

d. The method is a form of the continuity equation.

e. The method provides estimation of mitral valve area within 24 hours following mitral valvuloplasty.

Q8.5 All of the following can cause diastolic mitral regurgitation *except*:

a. Aortic regurgitation

b. Complete heart block

c. 1° atrioventricular block

d. Flail mitral leaflet

e. Constrictive pericarditis

Q8.6 The mitral valve area of a patient with rheumatic deformity is measured by PISA. The aliasing radius is 1 cm, the aliasing velocity is 30 cm/sec, the angle between the valve tips is 120°, and the peak mitral inflow velocity is 1.5 m/sec. What is the estimated mitral valve area?

a. 0.8 cm^2

b. 1.0 cm^2

c. 1.2 cm^2

d. 1.4 cm^2

e. 1.6 cm^2

Q8.7   The Doppler tracings shown in Figure Q8.7 demonstrate a series of Doppler mitral flows in a patient with mitral stenosis and atrial fibrillation. Which deceleration time has been measured properly?

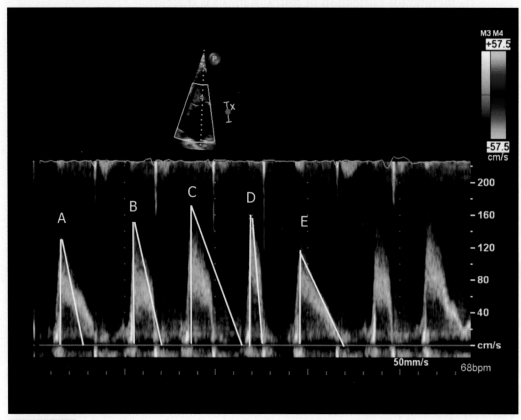

Figure Q8.7

a.   A = 336 msec

b.   B = 265msec

c.   C = 608 msec

d.   D = 142 msec

e.   E = 594 msec

Q8.8   Using the answer in the previous question, what is the estimated mitral valve area?

    a. $0.9\ cm^2$

    b. $1.1\ cm^2$

    c. $1.3\ cm^2$

    d. $1.5\ cm^2$

    e. $1.7\ cm^2$

Q8.9   If all of the deceleration times had been measured accurately in the Doppler tracings shown in Figure Q8.7, the average of how many beats would be required to produce an accurate estimate of mitral valve area?

    a.   1

    b.   2

    c.   3

    d.   4

    e.   5

Q8.10   Which of the following findings is a secondary sign of severe mitral regurgitation?

    a.   E to A reversal

    b.   Diminished diastolic pulmonary vein inflow

    c.   A restrictive pattern of mitral valve inflow

    d.   Right atrial enlargement

    e.   Reduced E′

Q8.11   Which of the following statements about PISA is accurate?

a. It is useful for determining the prognosis in patients with aortic regurgitation.

b. It uses flow *only* measured by pulse Doppler.

c. It is obtained from the parasternal views for estimation of ERO in patients with mitral regurgitation.

d. It uses the continuity equation to determine effective orifice area in patients with mitral regurgitation, aortic regurgitation, and mitral stenosis.

e. It cannot be used if regurgitation is present in the adjacent upstream or downstream valve.

ANSWERS

Q8.4 a: Decreased LV compliance increases the rate at which LA and LV pressures equilibrate, shortening the pressure half-time and producing an overestimation of mitral valve area. When aortic regurgitation is significant enough to raise LVEDP, it produces the same effect. (Section **8.4**)

Q8.5 d: Although complete heart block is the most notable cause of diastolic mitral regurgitation, any degree of atrioventricular block may produce the phenomenon. Other etiologies include premature ventricular beats, constrictive pericarditis, or an abrupt rise in LVEDP due to acute aortic regurgitation (Section **8.17**)

Q8.6 a: ERO by PISA is calculated as follows:

$$\frac{(6.28)(\text{PISA radius})(\text{aliasing velocity})(\text{angle between valve tips}/180°)}{\text{MV inflow velocity}}$$

$$= \frac{(6.28)(1 \text{ cm}^2)(30 \text{ cm/sec})}{150 \text{ cm/sec}} \times \frac{120}{180}$$

$$= 0.84 \text{ cm}^2$$

(Section **8.5**)

Q8.7 e: If the initial deceleration across the mitral valve decreases, the most accurate result will be obtained by using the shallower slope. (Section **8.4**)

Q8.8 c

$$\text{mitral valve area} = 750/\text{deceleration time} = 750/594 = 1.3 \text{ cm}^2$$

or

$$\text{mitral valve area} = \frac{220}{(0.29)(\text{deceleration time})}$$

$$= \frac{220}{(0.29)(594)}$$

$$= 1.3 \text{ cm}^2$$

(Section **8.4**)

Q8.9 e: In the presence of atrial fibrillation, at least five consecutive beats are recommended for accurate estimation of either mitral or aortic valve area. (Section **8.4**)

Q8.10   c: Severe mitral regurgitation can produce a shortened deceleration time as the result of the elevation in left atrial pressure. (Section **8.13**)

Q8.11   d: PISA is a form of the continuity equation and can be used in all the settings described in this answer. It provides important prognostic information in patients with mitral regurgitation. It requires both color-flow and CW Doppler for estimation of valve area. For calculation of ERO in mitral regurgitation, apical views are necessary. As with any continuity equation measure, adjacent valvular regurgitation will not affect its accuracy. (Section **8.15**)

THE RIGHT HEART AND PULMONARY HYPERTENSION

Q9.1 The M-mode echocardiogram through the pulmonic valve demonstrates (Figure Q9.1):

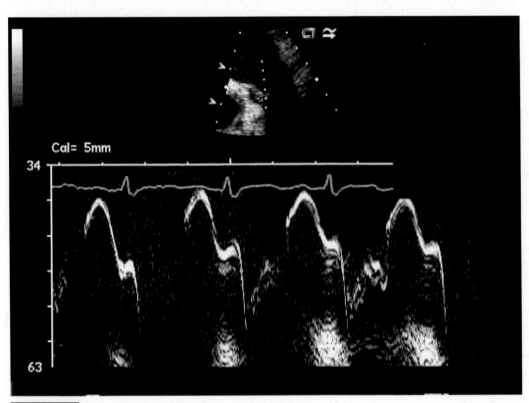

Figure Q9.1

a. Pulmonic stenosis

b. Pulmonic regurgitation

c. Pulmonary hypertension

d. RV failure

e. Constrictive pericarditis

Q9.2   In the setting of pulmonary artery hypertension, which of the following echocardiographic findings is an independent predictor of survival?

a. RV stroke volume

b. Tricuspid regurgitation jet width

c. RV hypokinesis with apical sparing (McConnell sign)

d. Diastolic hepatic vein flow reversal

e. Tricuspid annular plane displacement

Q9.3   An 18-year-girl is referred for TTE after two episodes of syncope. The LV is normal. The RV demonstrates RVOT dilation, free wall sacculations, and a thickened moderator band. The most likely diagnosis is:

a. Uhl's anomaly (parchment right ventricle)

b. Brugada syndrome

c. Arrythmogenic right ventricular cardiomyopathy

d. Scleroderma

e. Fabry disease

ANSWERS: 9.1. c; 9.2. e; 9.3. c

9.1   *Normal measures of RV size and function*: The RV is a challenging chamber to image by 2D echocardiography. Because of its crescent shape wrapping around the LV, RV volume is more difficult to measure, and RV systolic function can be equally difficult to quantify. Nevertheless, echocardiography plays an irreplaceable role in the evaluation of RV systolic function and its assessment in a variety of disease states.

Normal RV diameters are commonly measured from the apical four-chamber view at the base (normal diameter is 2.0–2.8 cm) and midlevel (normal diameter is 2.7–3.3 cm). The RVOT diameter is measured in parasternal short axis view (normal is 2.5–2.9 cm above the aortic valve and 1.7–2.3 cm above pulmonary artery). Normal base-to-apex length from the four-chamber view is 7.1–7.9 cm.

9.2   *RV systolic dysfunction* from any cause produces characteristic findings. RV dilation may be seen in either apical or subcostal views. The pattern of dilation may provide soft clues to the diagnosis, as in arrythmogenic RV cardiomyopathy or pulmonary embolism. *Diastolic septal flattening* occurs as the result of volume overload, (as seen with an atrial septal defect or severe tricuspid regurgitation) and, consequently, elevated RV diastolic pressure. When RV volume is sufficiently elevated, the interventricular septum shifts toward the LV in diastole but then rounds back to normal in systole as LV systolic pressure rises normally above RV systolic pressure. If RV systolic pressure is markedly elevated, septal flattening will occur during systole (Figure 9.1).

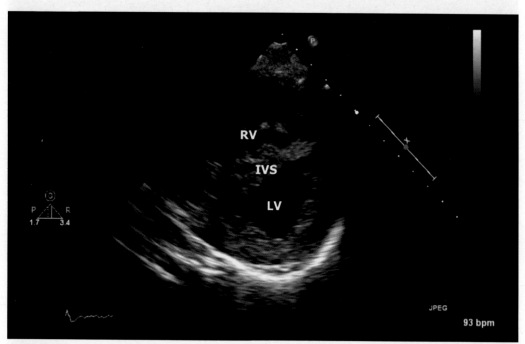

Figure 9.1   TTE parasternal short axis. Interventricular diastolic septal flattening is secondary to RV volume load. IVS, interventricular septum.

LEARNING DIRECTIVE

See Clip 9.2: Septal flattening throughout the cardiac cycle characteristic of combined RV volume and pressure overload.

The close correlate of this sign is *paradoxical septal motion*, also a sign of excess RV volume overload. The increased RV volume increases RV contractility with the resultant movement of the septum toward the RV as the entire LV is displaced anteriorly toward the transducer (Figure 9.2). Other causes of paradoxical septal motion include prior cardiac surgery and left bundle branch block.

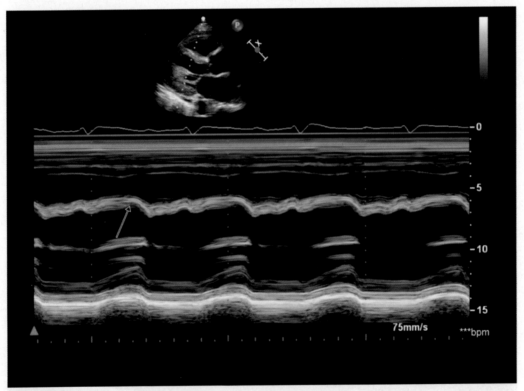

Figure 9.2 The M-mode appearance of paradoxical systolic septal motion (arrow) secondary to RV pressure overload.

LEARNING DIRECTIVE

See Clip 9.3: Paradoxical septal motion produced by RV volume overload.

9.3.   *RVOT acceleration time (AcT) (Mahan equation)*: The AcT is the time from onset of pulmonary flow to the peak of the RVOT VTI (Figure 9.3).

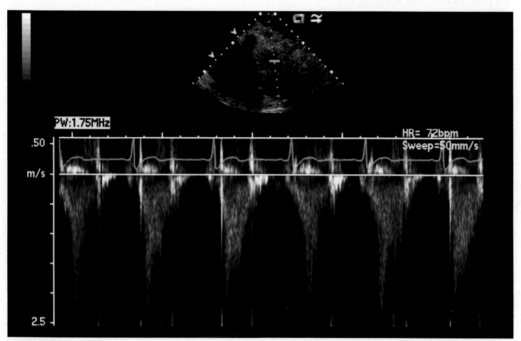

Figure 9.3   AcT is shortened in this patient with pulmonary hypertension.

The Mahan equation uses the AcT to estimate mean pulmonary artery pressure according to the following formula:

$$\text{mean PA pressure} = 79 - 0.45(\text{AcT})$$

Note that the shorter the AcT, the higher the mean pulmonary artery pressure and that an AcT of 50 produces a mean pulmonary artery pressure of about 55 mm Hg.

9.4   *Pulmonary vascular resistance (PVR)* can be estimated by substituting Doppler-based estimates of right heart pressures into the classic formula in the following manner:

$$\text{PVR} = \frac{(\text{mean PA pressure} - \text{wedge pressure})}{\text{cardiac output}}$$

This equation translates to:

$$\text{PVR} = 10 \times \frac{\text{TR jet velocity}}{\text{RVOT}_{\text{VTI}}} + 0.16$$

The equation uses the tricuspid regurgitation jet in units of m/sec and the RVOT in cm.

As an example, given a tricuspid regurgitant jet peak velocity of 3 m/sec and RVOT VTI of 19 cm, the PVR is:

$$10 \times \frac{3.0}{19} + 0.16 = 1.7 \text{ woods units}$$

Tricuspid annular displacement, or tricuspid annular plane systolic excursion (TAPSE), is a measure of RV systolic function that simply determines the apical displacement of the tricuspid annulus in systole. Normal is > 16 mm. Studies have reported an association using this index between pulmonary artery systolic hypertension and decreased survival.

9.5   In the absence of pulmonic stenosis, pulmonary artery systolic pressure equals RV systolic pressure and is easily measured using the tricuspid regurgitant peak velocity as described in the Doppler section. To estimate RA pressure, measure the IVC *diameter and its response to respiration* (Table 9.1).

Table 9.1 IVC Diameter and Associated Findings

IVC Diameter	Respiratory Collapse	Estimated RA Pressure
< 2.1 cm	> 50%	≤ 5 mm Hg
> 2.1 cm	< 50%	≥ 15 mm Hg
Intermediate states no fulfilling either of the above criteria:		5–15 mm Hg

Tricuspid Regurgitation

9.6   Although a few conditions cause intrinsic tricuspid valve disease (i.e., endocarditis, carcinoid disease, rheumatic heart disease), most tricuspid regurgitation is functional. The valve leaks either because the pressure in the RV has risen for some other reason, such as lung disease, pulmonary embolism, or RV infarction, or the geometry of the RV is altered by a similar set of causes.

9.7   *Criteria for severe tricuspid regurgitation:*

1. The dagger sign: a dense spectral Doppler jet that ends in a peak with a concave or "dagger" configuration (Figure 9.4). Broad low-velocity flow jets can also be seen.

2. Hepatic vein flow reversal

LEARNING DIRECTIVE

See Clip 9.14: Hepatic vein flow reversal with respiration (the faint red flow), a hallmark of severe tricuspid regurgitation.

3. Tricuspid inflow velocity ≥ 1 m/sec

4. Tricuspid ERO ≥ 0.4 cm^2

5. $\dfrac{\text{TR jet area}}{\text{RA area}} > 30\%$

6. Annulus dilation > 4 cm

7. Tricuspid regurgitant volume ≥ 45 cc

8. Vena contracta width ≥ 6 mm

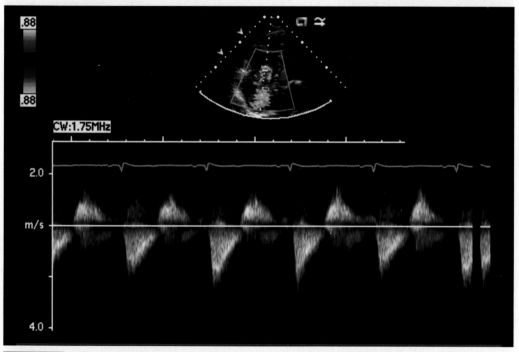

Figure 9.4   The spectral Doppler appearance of severe tricuspid regurgitation. Note the dagger-like shape of the jet.

Right Ventricular Echocardiographic Findings in Specific Disease States

9.8   *McConnell sign*: Pulmonary embolism may produce severe RV dilation with markedly decreased contraction with apical sparing (Figure 9.5). The RV apex contracts because LV function is unaffected with the RV apex pulled with the LV apex. In the absence of any previous injury or pulmonary hypertension, RV systolic pressure in this setting will usually rise to a maximum of approximately 50 mm Hg.

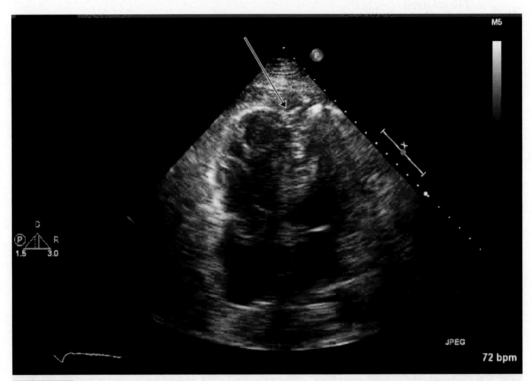

Figure 9.5   TTE apical four-chamber view showing the McConnell sign. RV dilation is present, but apical contraction (arrow) is preserved.

LEARNING DIRECTIVE

See Clip 9.9: Severe RV dilation and hypokinesis with apical sparing (McConnell sign). This finding is highly suggestive (but not diagnostic) of acute pulmonary embolism.

In contrast, pulmonary artery pressure in the setting of *RV infarction* will not rise, and may even be reduced depending upon volume status, because the ability of the RV to generate a pressure head is compromised. Under these circumstances, RV dysfunction may be generalized or focal, and a concomitant inferior or inferolateral LV wall motion abnormality will usually be seen.

9.9   *Arrhythmogenic right ventricular cardiomyopathy (ARVC)* (Figure 9.6): Multiple imaging modalities may be employed for identification or confirmation of the diagnosis. Echocardiography reveals several typical findings, including dilation of the RV and RVOT, RV free wall sacculations, and apical aneurysm.

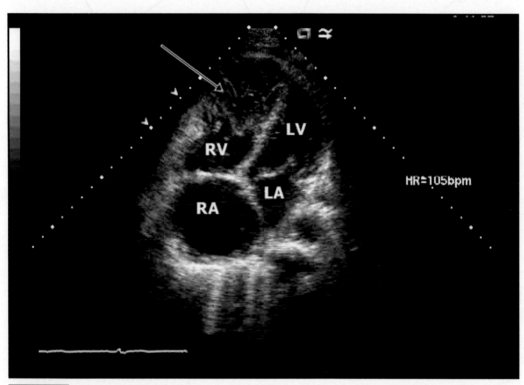

Figure 9.6   Arrhythmogenic RV cardiomyopathy. This apical four-chamber view was deliberately obtained off axis to accentuate the RV free wall. Note the intense trabeculations (arrow) at the apex.

Echocardiographic Signs of Pulmonary Artery Hypertension

9.10 When pulmonary artery pressure is normal, the M-mode tracing of the pulmonic valve produces a characteristic pattern, beginning with a small dip or A wave in late diastole as the result of atrial contraction, followed by gentle descent of the M-mode tracing through the posterior leaflet as the valve opens in systole under normal pressure (Figure 9.7).

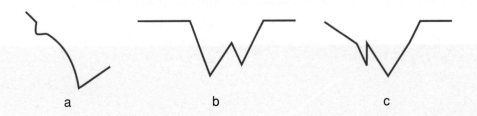

a   b   c

Figure 9.7   M-mode appearance of (a) a normal pulmonic valve, (b) a pulmonic valve in a patient with pulmonary artery hypertension, and (c) pulmonic valve stenosis.

In pulmonary artery hypertension, the A wave disappears because the effect produced by atrial contraction is masked by the increased pulmonary artery diastolic pressure. The descent of the posterior leaflet steepens and the tracing assumes a typical "W" shape as the rate of valve closure is increased by the elevated downstream pulmonary pressure. With pulmonic stenosis, the A wave reappears in a slightly accentuated form prior to pulmonic valve opening, and the slope of the tracing produced by pulmonic valve closure at end systole is once again steep because of the limited excursion of the valve. Midsystolic closure occurs as the rate of rise in RV pressure nears its apex, and the rate of ascent of the tracing is also accentuated by the rapid rate of valve closure.

The shape and magnitude of the pulmonic outflow VTI is altered by pulmonary hypertension in a similar fashion. Normal pulmonic flow velocity is ≤ 1.5 m/sec. An increase in the downward slope of the acceleration phase will reflect the decreased acceleration time (Figure 9.3). Systolic notching in the pulmonic valve VTI will reflect midsystolic closure (Figure 9.8) in the setting of severe pulmonic stenosis (Figure 9.9).

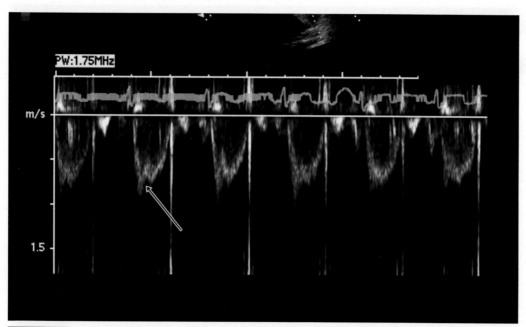

Figure 9.8   Spectral Doppler of PV outflow in pulmonic stenosis demonstrating midsystolic closure (arrow).

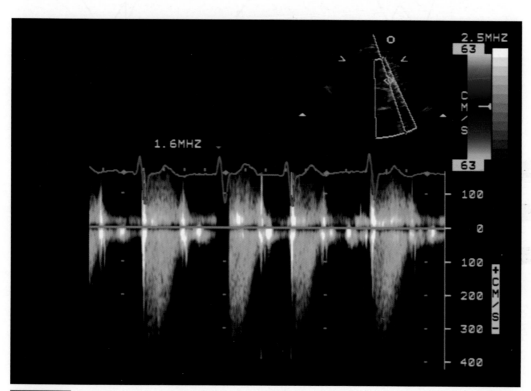

Figure 9.9   CW Doppler tracing across the RVOT in a patient with moderate to severe pulmonic stenosis (peak velocity = 3 m/sec).

ADVANCED QUESTIONS

Q9.4   Which two variables can be used to estimate pulmonary vascular resistance?

   a. Tricuspid regurgitant flow velocity and RVOT VTI

   b. Tricuspid inflow velocity and pulmonic regurgitation VTI

   c. IVC diameter and hepatic vein flow velocity

   d. TAPSE and RV inflow diameter

   e. Pulmonary vascular resistance cannot be estimated noninvasively.

For Questions 9.5–9.7, match the M-mode pulmonic valve tracing shown in Figure Q9.5 with the hemodynamic condition:

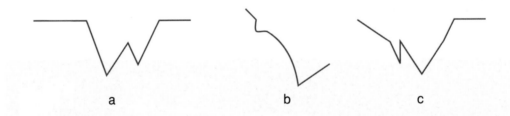

a   b   c

Figure Q9.5

Q9.5   Normal PA pressure

Q9.6   Pulmonary artery hypertension

Q9.7   Pulmonic valve stenosis

ANSWERS

Q9.4   a: The Doppler-derived equation for pulmonary vascular resistance is:

$$PVR = 10 \times \frac{TR \text{ jet velocity}}{VTI_{RVOT}} + 0.16$$

(Section **9.4**)

Q9.5   b: See Section **9.10** for answers to Q9.5–Q9.7.

Q9.6   a

Q9.7   c

Q10.1 Which statement about the image shown in Figure Q10.1 is correct?

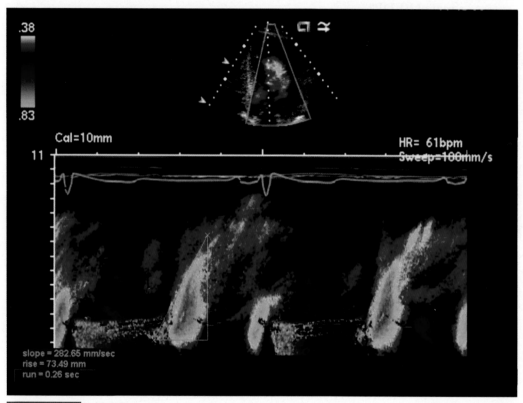

Figure Q10.1

    a.   The sample volume is placed in the LV apex.

    b.   A value < 25 cm/sec is normal.

    c.   The slope increases (gets faster) as diastolic dysfunction decreases.

    d.   The variable is measured using color-flow Doppler.

    e.   The variable displayed can be correlated to LVEDP.

Q10.2   Restrictive physiology demonstrates which of the following findings?

     a.   Loss of the systolic component of pulmonary venous inflow

     b.   Respiratory variation of mitral inflow

     c.   Prolonged isovolumic relaxation time

     d.   Transmitral Doppler E/A ratio > 1

     e.   Diastolic hepatic vein flow reversal

Q10.3   Which of the following variables *cannot* be combined to accurately estimate LVEDP?

     a.   Mitral E wave flow velocity and E' TDI (E/E')

     b.   End-diastolic aortic regurgitant flow velocity and diastolic blood pressure

     c. $-dP/dt$ and peak diastolic pulmonary flow

     d.   Transmitral Doppler E/A ratio and isovolumic relaxation

     e.   Pulmonary venous A-wave width and mitral A-wave width

ANSWERS: 10.1. e; 10.2. a; 10.3. c

10.1   Diastolic function remains among the most difficult practical problems in echocardiography, if not all of cardiology. The challenge is that two separate but related processes take place simultaneously in a highly coordinated fashion. The first process, intrinsic relaxation, is a load-independent, energy-requiring process in which actin-myosin bonds are actively broken, sarcomeres lengthen, and LV pressure falls. William Grossman, one of the pioneers in this field, would tell his fellows an amusing but instructive story about a colleague who worked with isolated rat hearts. The researcher would dump the explanted heart in a bucket of perfusate so that it would remain viable as he prepared his experiments, and he noticed that the rat heart would move around the bucket in a pulsatile fashion like a little motorboat. The correct inference that the investigator made from this finding was that a normal ventricle would fill even in the absence of a pressure gradient, because without such filling, the resultant systolic contraction would never propel the heart around the bucket!

10.2   The intrinsically generated drop in ventricular diastolic pressure segues into the second process, ventricular filling, which is a direct function of the atrioventricular pressure gradient. The rate of filling depends not only upon the rate at which ventricular relaxation occurs, but upon the LA pressure throughout diastole. LA pressure in turn is influenced by a variety of normal and abnormal factors. Its rise can be inferred by a variety of echocardiography findings, and it serves as a critical indicator of advancing diastolic dysfunction.

The Four Doppler-Derived Parameters That Describe Normal Diastolic Function

10.3   *Mitral valve inflow patterns, or the transmitral doppler E and A waves:* By convention, the pulse Doppler sample volume is placed at the *tips of the mitral leaflets in the open position*, where the orifice is small and flow velocities will be maximal. With normal diastolic function, peak E velocity is greater than peak A velocity, and the E/A ratio is > 1. The LV relaxes, diastolic pressure remains low, and compliance (dV/dP) is relatively high. Because most normal LV filling takes place during the passive filling phase, the contribution of LA contraction is low and the A wave is small. However, in a young, healthy patient, such as the one described in Figure 10.1, the normal deceleration time can be quite short (< 140 msec).

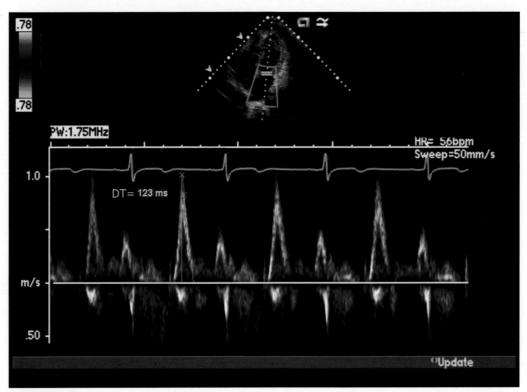

Figure 10.1   Transmitral inflow in a young, healthy adult may mimic a restrictive pattern. Note the short deceleration time (DT) of 123 msec.

10.4   *Timing intervals* include deceleration time, or DT (also discussed briefly in Section **8.4**), and isovolumic relaxation time (IVRT). Normal E-wave deceleration time is *140–220 msec*. Normal IVRT is *70–90 msec*. Deceleration time has both load-independent and dependent phases because it measures the rate of fall in diastolic pressure using the slope of the E wave. *IVRT lengthens with abnormal intrinsic relaxation, shortens with restriction, and demonstrates respiratory dependence in constriction.*

10.5   *Pulmonary (and systemic) vein flow patterns* consist of a biphasic systolic phase (PV_{s1} and PV_{s2}), a diastolic phase (PV_d), and an atrial flow reversal phase (PV_a) (Figure 10.2). Normal values are not usually assigned to these flows, but a normal ratio is $PV_{s2} \geq PV_d$. PV_{s1} occurs during *atrial relaxation*. PV_{s2} occurs during the atrial reservoir phase as venous blood fills the atrium. PV_d occurs during the conduit phase and reflects the atrioventricular pressure gradient. PV_a is the backflow wave created by active atrial contraction.

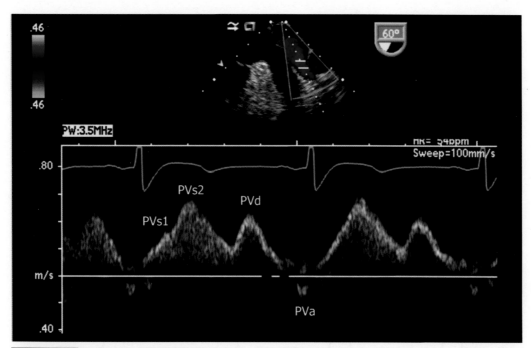

Figure 10.2   TEE midesophageal view of the normal pulmonary vein inflow pattern demonstrating all four phases.

10.6   *Tissue Doppler flow patterns,* diastolically speaking, include E′ and A′. In similar fashion to mitral inflow velocities, the normal pattern is E′ > A′.

Here is where it gets complicated (Figure 10.3).

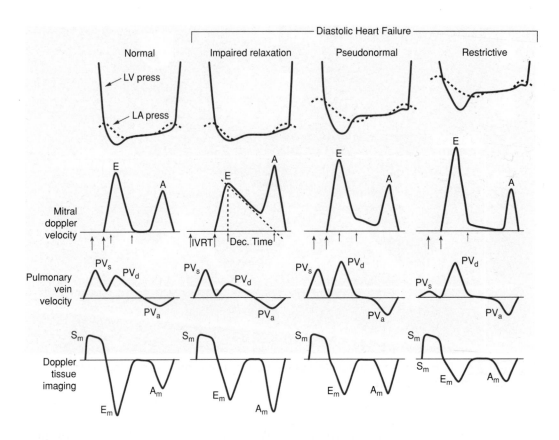

Figure 10.3   Stages of diastolic dysfunction. *Source*: Reprinted with permission from Zile MR. New Concepts in Diastolic Dysfunction and Diastolic Heart Failure: Part I: Diagnosis, Prognosis, and Measurements of Diastolic Function. *Circulation*. 2002;104:11.

The Three Stages of Diastolic Dysfunction According to Current Thinking

10.7 *Impaired relaxation*: In this phase, the intrinsic ability of the LV to relax is abnormal (often as the result of LV hypertrophy), though LA pressure is not elevated. Passive filling is impaired and the height of the transmitral E wave is shortened, but the increased rate of rise in LVEDP is modest. Consequently:

1. LA volume at the end of passive filling is increased, and the height of the transmitral A wave is increased, producing an E-to-A reversal or an E/A ratio < 1.

2. Because the rate of passive filling is also slowed, deceleration time increases.

3. Because pulmonary vein flow is dependent upon blood leaving the atrium and entering the ventricles and systolic filling is impaired, PV_d is decreased relative to PV_s.

4. Finally, TDIs show a corresponding reversal of E′ to A′, or an E′/A′ ratio > 1.

The trouble with this paradigm is that normal aging also leads to E-to-A reversal and a decline in E′ without diastolic dysfunction. Our advice, therefore, is that there should be at least two signs of diastolic dysfunction before you make this diagnosis. The ancillary findings of LV hypertrophy and/or LA enlargement are not specific, but they strengthen the certainty of diagnosis.

10.8 *Pseudonormalization* (Figure 10.4): In this more advanced phase, the degree of impaired relaxation has become more severe and has resulted in a faster, shorter, and incomplete filling phase, and a corresponding increase in LA pressure. As a result, E-wave velocity increases, deceleration time shortens, and E/A ratio once again becomes > 1 as it pseudonormalizes.

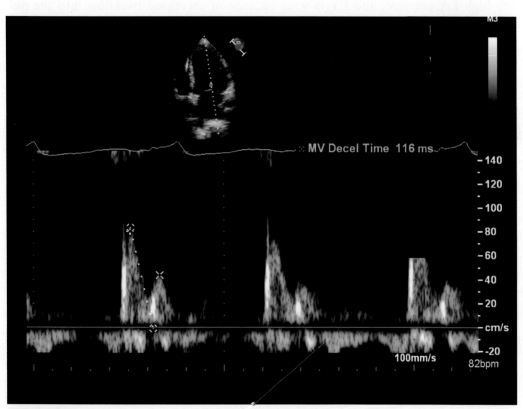

Figure 10.4 Transmitral Doppler example of pseudonormalization. Note the normal E/A ratio. The deceleration time (116 msec), however, is short.

PV_d rises and PV_s falls because whatever blood gets into the LA does so in diastole; PV_a widens as the inability of LA contraction to propel blood into the LA results in a longer, larger reversal of pulmonary vein flow.

A good test to distinguish pseudonormal from normal mitral inflow is the *Valsalva maneuver.* During a Valsalva, blood is excluded from the LA by the transient increase in intrathoracic pressure. The resultant decrease in LA pressure will produce a normalization of mitral inflow, the pseudonormal pattern will disappear, and E/A will *decrease.* A normal mitral inflow pattern is unchanged by Valsalva because LA pressure is normal to begin with. The TDI pattern follows the alteration in mitral inflow, with an increased E′ relative to A′.

10.9 *Restrictive physiology* is the final phase in the paradigm. Think of the ventricle in this condition as a rigid box with a finite volume. Any blood that is going to get in does so early in diastole. LA diastolic pressure rises rapidly because of the absence of ventricular compliance, producing a tall spike-like E wave with a short deceleration time. LA pressure is high and the ability of the LA to accept atrial filling is severely compromised, so the A wave is small and short. PV_s is markedly reduced because of the high LA pressure, and PV_a is wide because of increased backflow into the pulmonary vein. The ratio of PV_a width to A-wave width therefore is increased. Finally, diastolic TDIs are reduced.

Load-Independent Indices

10.10 *–dP/dt*: The rate of fall in diastolic pressure with time, –dP/dt, can be measured noninvasively in a patient with mitral regurgitation in the same fashion described previously; however, velocities and time intervals are measured on the other side of the mitral regurgitation jet. As with dP/dt, –dP/dt assesses intrinsic relaxation independent of loading conditions.

Tau (or τ) is the time constant of LV relaxation (fasten your mathematical seatbelt). Because LV diastolic pressure falls exponentially, its rate of fall can be expressed as an exponential function: $P_v = P_0(e^{-t/\tau})$, where P_v is the pressure at any point in time, P_0 is pressure at max –dP/dt, and t is time. If you solve this equation by taking the natural log of both sides (or plot the natural log of P vs. t), you get a linear expression in which tau is the slope at maximum –dP/dt. Like –dP/dt, tau is an intrinsic property of the diastolic function of any given heart and is not dependent on changes in loading conditions.

Tau is classically measured in the catheterization laboratory by plotting LV diastolic pressure against time and solving the exponential function at maximum –dP/dt, as previously described; however, it can also be measured noninvasively using the mitral regurgitation jet in a fashion similar to –dP/dt. For a given heart, tau is quite challenging to calculate, but it is a gold standard index against which any new load-independent noninvasive measure is compared. Thus you will frequently come across statements that such and such an index is "highly correlated to tau."

10.11 *Flow propagation velocity, or* V_p (although whether this parameter is really load independent has lately become more controversial) (Figure 10.5): V_p is derived by color M-mode as the slope of the tangent line produced by the blue color map of mitral inflow; the shallower the slope, the slower the rate of intrinsic relaxation. V_p correlates well with tau, the time constant of relaxation (see the previous section). A normal value is $\geq$ 50 cm/sec.

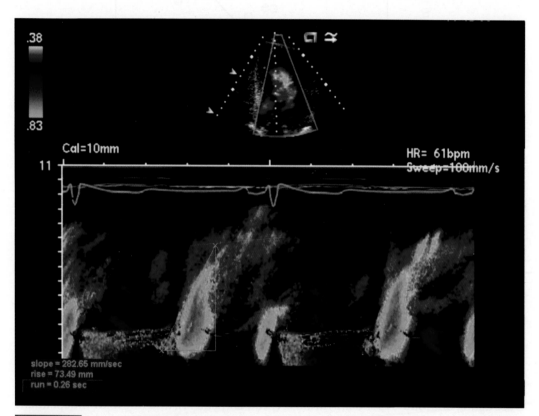

Figure 10.5   Flow propagation velocity V_p. A normal value is $\geq$ 50 cm/sec. In this patient, a the reduced value of 28 cm/sec is consistent with abnormal relaxation.

10.12 *Indices of filling pressures* frequently combine one load-independent variable and one load-dependent variable.

The E/E' ratio is linearly related to LVEDP, assuming LV systolic function is normal (Figure 10.6). The relationship is particularly informative at its extremes, such that an E/E' ratio $\leq$ 8 predicts a pulmonary capillary wedge pressure of < 12 mm Hg, and an

E/E′ > 15 predicts a pulmonary capillary wedge pressure of > 18 mm Hg. More recent data, however, suggest that the relationship breaks down in the presence of significant systolic dysfunction.

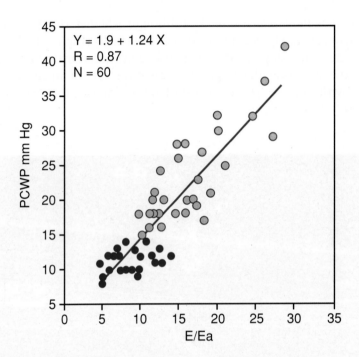

Figure 10.6   The relation between E/E′ and LV end-diastolic pressure. *Source*: From Nagueh. *JACC* 1997:1527–1533. Used with permission.

In a similar fashion, the product of peak E velocity multiplied by peak A velocity can be combined with IVRT. In congestive heart failure:

mean pulmonary capillary wedge pressure = 17 + (5.3)(peak E)(peak A) − (11)(IVRT)

Once again, one load-dependent variable, (peak E)(peak A), and one load-independent variable, IVRT, are combined, in this case to noninvasively calculate wedge pressure.

ADVANCED QUESTIONS

Q10.4   What clinical maneuver has occurred between the two spectral Doppler
tracings shown in Figure Q10.4?

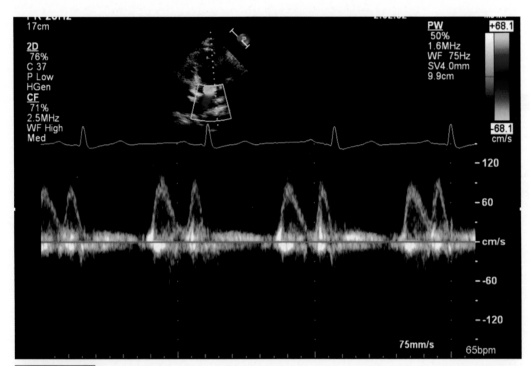

Figure Q10.4a

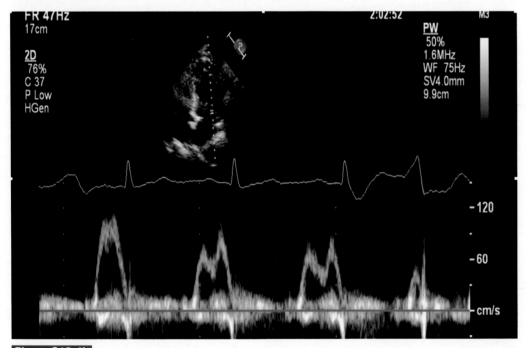

Figure Q10.4b

a. Inspiration

b. Expiration

c. Handgrip

d. Straight leg raising

e. Valsalva

Q10.5 A decrease in the normal rate of LV relaxation during diastole will:

a. Produce an underestimation of the mitral valve area using the pressure half-time method

b. Produce an overestimation of the mitral valve area using the pressure half-time method

c. Produce an underestimation of the aortic valve area using the continuity equation

d. Produce an overestimation of the aortic valve area using the continuity equation

e. Have no effect upon estimation of mitral valve area or aortic valve area

For Questions 10.6–10.9, match the letter in Figure Q10.6 with the correct description.

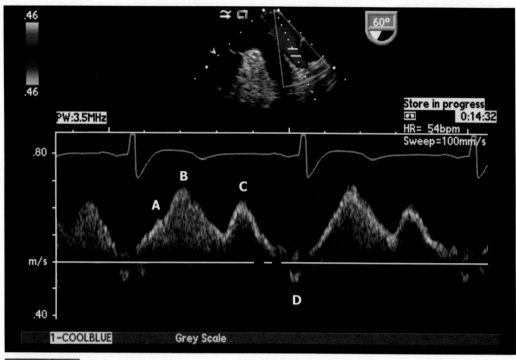

Figure Q10.6

Q10.6   Increases in width as LA pressure rises

Q10.7   Describes the rate and extent of LA relaxation

Q10.8   Decreases in height as LA pressure rises

Q10.9   Decreases in height as LA compliance decreases, but LA pressure remains normal

ANSWERS

Q10.4   e: This is a nice example of pseudonormalization of mitral inflow revealed through the Valsalva maneuver. (Section **10.8**)

Q10.5   b: See Section **8.4**.

Q10.6   d: PV_a widens as LA pressure increases, causing the ratio of PV_a to A to increase. (Section **10.9**)

Q10.7   a: PV_{s1} is due to atrial filling cause by atrial relaxation. (Section **10.5**)

Q10.8   b: PV_s falls during the restrictive phase of diastolic dysfunction. (Section **10.9**)

Q10.9   c: PV_d declines during the early phase of diastolic dysfunction, during which LA pressure is still relatively normal. (Section **10.7**)

PRACTICE QUESTIONS

Q11.1   What hemodynamic parameter is most commonly elevated in patients who demonstrate the abnormality shown in this M-mode echocardiogram?

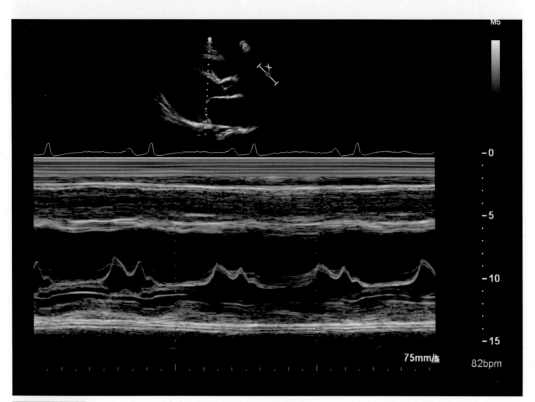

Figure Q11.1

    a.   LV end-diastolic volume

    b.   LV end-diastolic pressure

    c.   RV end-diastolic pressure

    d.   Pulmonary artery diastolic pressure

    e.   Pulmonary artery systolic pressure

Q11.2   What hemodynamic parameter is most commonly elevated in patients who demonstrate the abnormality shown in the M-mode echocardiogram in Figure Q11.2?

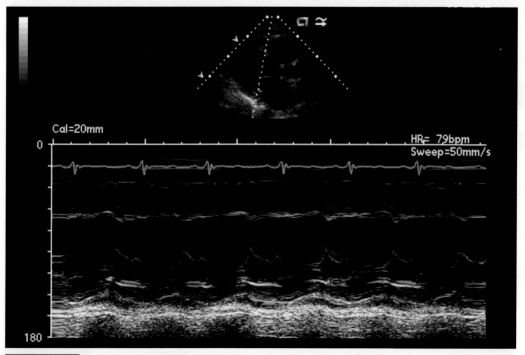

Figure Q11.2

a. LV end-diastolic volume

b. LV end-diastolic pressure

c. RV end-diastolic pressure

d. Pulmonary artery diastolic pressure

e. Pulmonary artery systolic pressure

Q11.3 You are asked to estimate the aortic valve area in a patient with known hypertrophic obstructive cardiomyopathy. The peak velocity in the distal LVOT by PW Doppler interrogation is 2 m/sec. The peak velocity in the proximal LVOT produces aliasing. The peak velocity across the entire LVOT detected by CW Doppler interrogation is 5 m/sec. The estimated gradient across the aortic valve is:

a. 16 mm Hg

b. 48 mm Hg

c. 109 mm Hg

d. 125 mm Hg

e. It cannot be determined from the information provided.

ANSWERS: 11.1. b; 11.2. a; 11.3. e

11.1 Echocardiography readily aids in the standard classification of cardiomyopathy into its three common subtypes. Both end-diastolic and end-systolic volumes are increased in the presence of *dilated cardiomyopathy*, and ejection fraction may be reduced across a broad range of values. As LV volume increases, ventricular geometry assumes a more spherical shape and the ratio of length to short axis diameter, or *sphericity index*, falls from a normal value of greater than 1.5 toward 1.0. Focal wall motion abnormalities may be seen even in the absence of ischemic heart disease, as in patients with acute myocarditis, or LV systolic dysfunction may be global, although the inferolateral wall will often be spared. Even in the presence of coronary artery disease or previous myocardial infarction, specific wall motion abnormalities become difficult to detect below an ejection fraction of 20%.

LV dysfunction may present with or without RV involvement. As LV dilation increases, the mitral annulus becomes dilated and mitral regurgitation becomes increasingly common, even in the absence of intrinsic valvular abnormalities. This circumstance in turn may contribute to progression of LV dilation. Intracavitary thrombus, often at the apex, may also be seen, especially with the use of a contrast agent such as perflutren (Definity™). At the advanced stage, spectral Doppler demonstrates secondary restrictive filling abnormalities with transmitral E-to-A reversal, shortened deceleration time and increased E/E′ ratio. When present, a restrictive filling pattern is a marker of decreased survival independent of systolic function.

11.2 Two longstanding and still useful M-mode signs of LV systolic dysfunction bear mentioning. Elevated LVEDP may produce a slight delay in systolic closure of the mitral valve resulting in a characteristic "*B bump*" in the anterior mitral leaflet just after the mitral A wave (Figure Q11.1). Elevated LV diastolic volume will manifest as a broad separation between the E wave and the septum, or *E-point septal separation* (Figure Q11.2).

11.3 Several morphologic subtypes of dilated cardiomyopathy can be readily identified by echocardiography. *Takotsubo cardiomyopathy of the LV*, or apical ballooning, classically produces a pattern of severe dilation of the apical two-thirds of the LV with preserved basal function (Figure 11.1). Diffuse ST elevation is often present, but coronary angiography demonstrates minimal or no luminal disease. Thought to be secondary to catecholamine surge in the setting of a physical or emotional insult ("broken heart syndrome"), Takotsubo cardiomyopathy usually improves spontaneously or resolves within 1 to 4 weeks. Apical thrombus may form in the acute phase.

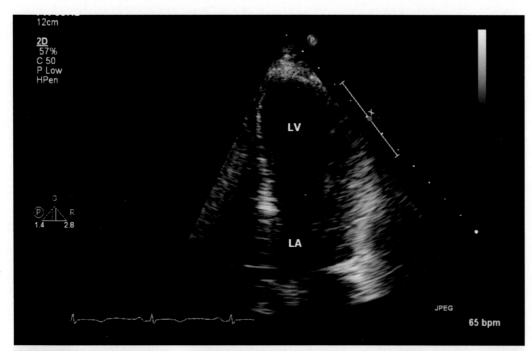

Figure 11.1 TTE in the apical four-chamber view in a patient with Takotsubo cardiomyopathy. Note the dilated apex.

LEARNING DIRECTIVE

See Clip 11.3: Takotsubo cardiomyopathy seen in the four-chamber view. Note the apical ballooning.

11.4 *Ventricular noncompaction* is a congenital anomaly caused by embryonic failure of cardiac muscle fibers to assemble and compress properly. It is characterized by deep crevices with the myocardial wall, especially involving the LV apex, with a ratio of compacted to noncompacted tissue of > 1.7 to 1 (Figure 11.2). The condition most often presents as heart failure among patients in early middle age. As a rule, LV systolic function is significantly decreased and prognosis is guarded. LV thrombus and arrhythmias are common.

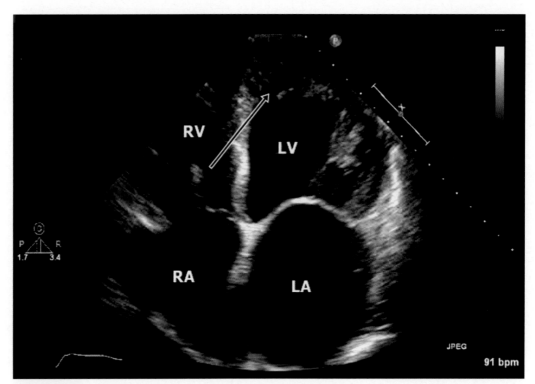

Figure 11.2   TTE in the apical four-chamber view in a patient with ventricular noncompaction. Note the deep endocardial crevices (arrow).

LEARNING DIRECTIVE

See Clip 11.6: LV noncompaction seen in the four-chamber view. Note the deep crevices in the distal portion of the ventricle.

11.5   *Hypertrophic nonobstructive cardiomyopathy* (HCM) presents as markedly increased LV wall thickness ($\geq$ 15 mm), the absence of hypertension or aortic stenosis, normal or small LV cavity, and normal regional and global systolic function, with varying degrees of diastolic dysfunction and increased LA volume. Even in the setting of mild or well-controlled hypertension, an elevated LV mass index is a marker of likelihood of progression to heart failure, development of atrial fibrillation, and reduced survival.

11.6   *Hypertrophic obstructive cardiomyopathy* (HOCM) is a disease that cardiologist and echocardiographer alike appreciate because its pathology exemplifies so many basic principles of cardiac hemodynamics. Although the degree of LVOT obstruction is a ready measure of disease severity, diastolic dysfunction is also a universal and clinically relevant finding. The echocardiographic hallmarks of HOCM include:

1.   *Systolic anterior motion of the mitral valve*: Long-term debate continues over whether this archetypal sign is a cause or consequence of LVOT obstruction. Either way, its presence provides a key criterion for the diagnosis, and it is readily identified by M-mode (Figure 11.3) as well as 2D echocardiography (Figure 11.4).

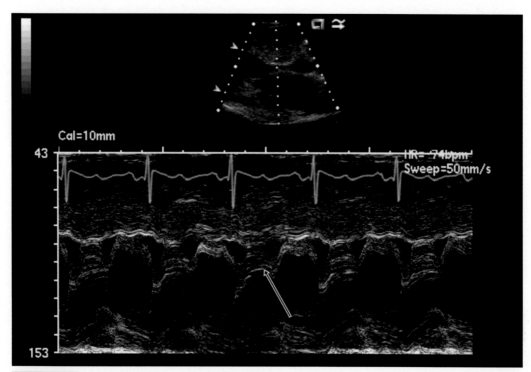

Figure 11.3 Hypertrophic obstructive cardiomyopathy with systolic anterior motion of the mitral valve demonstrated by M-mode (arrow).

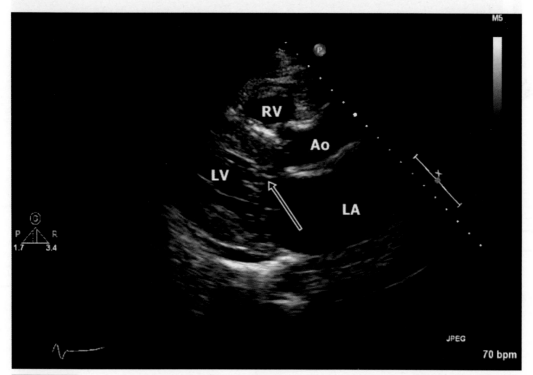

Figure 11.4 TTE parasternal long axis view in a patient with hypertrophic obstructive cardiomyopathy with systolic anterior motion (arrow) of the mitral valve leaflets.

See Clip 11.15: The 2D pattern of systolic anterior motion.

2. *Asymmetric septal hypertrophy*: The qualifying ratio for this condition is greater than 1.5 to 1 in the absence of infarction. Asymmetric basal septal thickening can also be found as a nonspecific and benign finding in elderly patients in the absence of other findings suggestive of obstruction. Though less common, focal hypertrophy can also be present elsewhere in both HCM and HOCM.

3. *LVOT gradients* (Figure 11.5): Depending upon the severity, there may be no gradient at rest and a gradient that is provocable with Valsalva or a significant resting gradient that increases with Valsalva. The gradient has a characteristic dagger-like shape secondary to the dynamic nature of the obstruction, in which the degree of obstruction increases as LV contractility increases throughout systole.

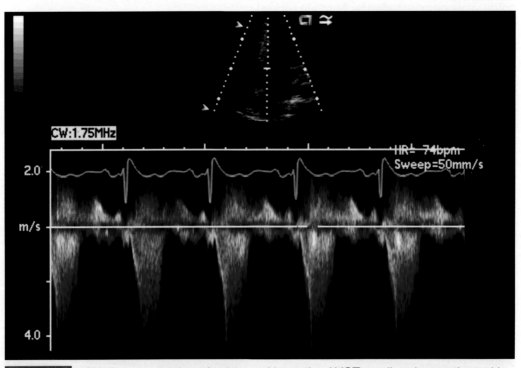

Figure 11.5   CW Doppler tracing of a 64 mm Hg resting LVOT gradient in a patient with hypertrophic obstructive cardiomyopathy.

The acceleration of the gradient also leads to a transient decline in outflow exemplified by *midsystolic closure of the aortic valve*, seen as a notching in the usual parallelogram shape of the aortic valve in systole on M-mode (Figure 11.6).

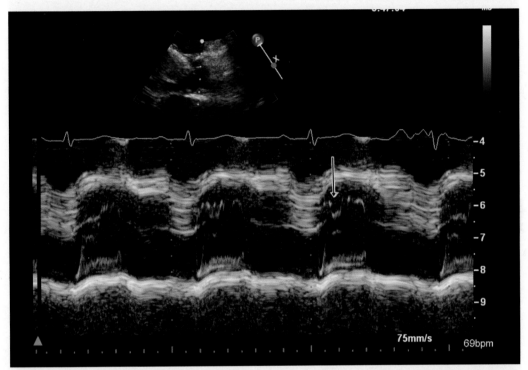

Figure 11.6   Midsystolic closure (arrow) of the aortic valve in a patient with hypertrophic obstructive cardiomyopathy.

4. *Mitral regurgitation* is a nearly universal feature of HOCM. The mitral regurgitation jet can be differentiated from the LVOT jet by its greater width, its initiation coincident with the onset of systole, and its symmetrical shape.

In severe HOCM, the prolonged relaxation phase may produce a third peak during mitral inflow that occurs just at the beginning of diastole and before mitral valve opening. This flow is referred to as *isovolumic relaxation flow* (Figure 11.7).

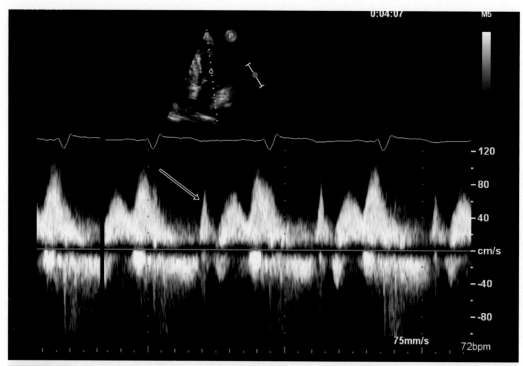

Figure 11.7   Isovolumic relaxation flow (arrow) secondary to impaired relaxation.

Echocardiography can be used to guide septal ablation therapy. Perflutren (Definity™) is injected in the first septal perforator to define its territory and ensure that the catheter is properly placed prior to injection of ethanol (Figure 11.8).

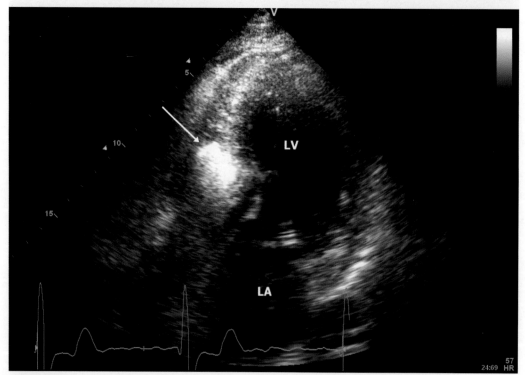

Figure 11.8   TTE four-chamber view demonstrates opacification of the intra-atrial septum (arrow) after injection of perflutren contrast into a catheter placed in the first septal perforator of the left anterior descending artery in preparation for ethanol ablation.

11.7 Other variants of HOCM include *apical hypertrophic cardiomyopathy* (Yamaguchi syndrome, or spade heart). Intracavitary gradients may be detected by Doppler interrogation, but there is no LVOT obstruction.

LEARNING DIRECTIVE

See Clip 11.20b: A typical example of apical hypertrophic cardiomyopathy (Yamaguchi syndrome, or spade heart). Note the apical cavity obliteration.

Restrictive Cardiomyopathy

11.8 The most common cause of restrictive cardiomyopathy in the U.S. population is *amyloid heart disease* in its late stages (Figure 11.9). The LV characteristically demonstrates marked symmetric thickening in the absence of ECG findings of hypertrophy with poor contraction. The RV is frequently dilated as the result of pulmonary hypertension.

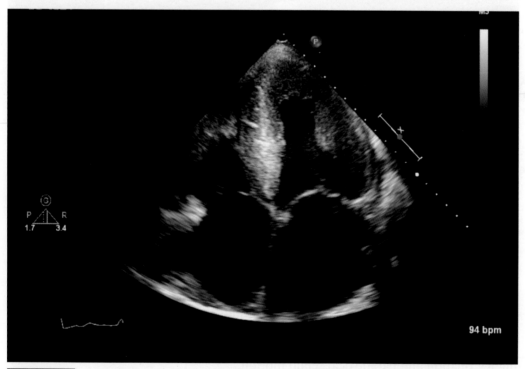

Figure 11.9   TTE apical four-chamber view in a patient with cardiac amyloidosis. Note the symmetrical LV wall thickening, bilateral atrial enlargement, and RV dilation.

At the advanced stage, hemodynamic findings typical for restriction include short deceleration time and IVRT, increased E/A, absent PV_s, and a wide PV_a. Respiratory variation of peak mitral inflow velocities is absent, and peak relaxation velocities measured by TDI are reduced.

Left Ventricular Assist Devices

11.9 A normally functioning ventricular assist device produces a characteristic series of echocardiographic findings. Blood flow is routed though the device, usually in the LV apex, to the aorta (Figure 11.10).

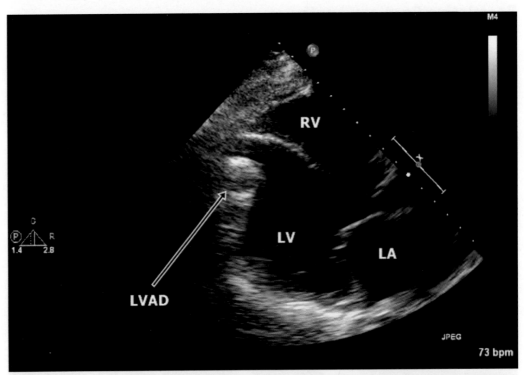

Figure 11.10   TTE parasternal long axis view in a patient with a left ventricular assist device (LVAD; arrow) placed in the LV apex.

When the device is functioning as intended, the aortic leaflets will remain closed (or nearly closed) throughout the cardiac cycle, and there will be minimal RV volume overload. By contrast, partial occlusion of the device leading to inadequate flow will force the aortic valve to open and may produce signs of RV volume overload, including RV dilation and paradoxical septal motion.

ADVANCED QUESTIONS

Q11.4 You are called to the surgical intensive care unit to perform an urgent TEE on a patient 12 hours after mechanical mitral valve replacement. The patient's systolic blood pressure is 90 mm Hg, and he is receiving near maximal doses of dopamine and norepinephrine. TEE demonstrates no mitral regurgitation and hyperdynamic LV systolic function. RV cavity size and systolic function are normal, and there is no pericardial effusion. Which of the following spectral Doppler gradients will most likely reveal the etiology of the patient's hypotension?

a. Maximal tricuspid regurgitation jet

b. Maximal LVOT gradient

c. Maximal mitral inflow gradient

d. Maximal pulmonic outflow gradient

e. Maximal pulmonary vein systolic gradient

Q11.5 You are asked to evaluate the function of an LV assist device at the bedside of a patient with advanced heart failure and persistent hypotension. Standard echocardiographic images from the parasternal long axis view reveal no opening of the aortic valve and mild aortic regurgitation. The LV is severely dilated and systolic function is severely reduced. The RV is normal in size but demonstrates severe systolic dysfunction. There is a small circumferential pericardial effusion without evidence of RA or RV diastolic collapse. There is no respiratory variation of mitral inflow by spectral Doppler imaging. The device is seen at the apex in the parasternal long axis views but not in the apical views.

a. The device is occluded.

b. The device is functioning normally.

c. The device is improperly placed.

d. The device is functioning properly, but the flow rate needs to be increased.

e. The device is infected.

Q11.6   The Doppler flow tracing in Figure Q11.6 is most characteristic of:

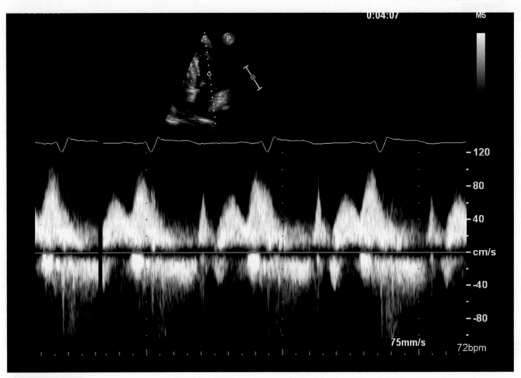

Figure Q11.6

a. Ischemic cardiomyopathy

b. Amyloid heart disease

c. Sarcoidosis

d. Severe hypertrophic obstructive cardiomyopathy

e. Severe pulmonary hypertension

Q11.7 The M-mode tracing in Figure Q11.7 demonstrates:

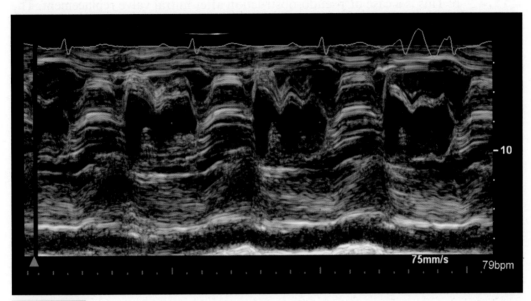

Figure Q11.7

a. Endocarditis

b. Asymmetrical septal hypertrophy

c. Flail mitral leaflet

d. Systolic anterior motion of the mitral valve leaflets.

e. Premature aortic valve closure

ANSWERS

Q11.4 b: This is a case of pseudo-obstruction after mitral valve replacement. The cause of hypotension is underfilling of the LV with protrusion of the new mitral prosthesis into the LVOT and a subsequent LVOT gradient. Once the LVOT gradient of 70 mm Hg was documented, the patient improved with fluid administration and discontinuation of pressors.

Q11.5 b: The description in the question is of a normally functioning LV assist device. The cause of this patient's hypotension is severe RV dysfunction, which is commonly seen in this setting. The device is often seen only in one imaging plane. (Section **11.9**)

Q11.6 d: The extra initial spike seen at the beginning of diastole is isovolumic relaxation flow, seen in the setting of HOCM when advanced diastolic dysfunction is present. (Section **11.6**)

Q11.7 d: See Section **11.6**.

12 CONGENITAL HEART DISEASE

David I. Silverman, Felice A. Heller, and Warren J. Manning

PRACTICE QUESTIONS

Q12.1 Which two types of ventricular septal defect are difficult to distinguish in the parasternal long axis view because of their similar location?

    a. Perimembranous and muscular

    b. Muscular and supracristal

    c. Supracristal and inlet

    d. Inlet and perimembranous

    e. Supracristal and perimembranous

Q12.2 Which alternative view is most useful for distinguishing the answer to Question 12.1?

    a. RV inflow

    b. Parasternal short axis

    c. Apical four-chamber

    d. Apical three-chamber

    e. Apical five-chamber

Q12.3   Injection of saline contrast produces full opacification of the RA within one beat, followed by an area of pulsatile clearing originating directly from the midinteratrial septum (negative contrast effect). The most likely diagnosis is:

a.   Patent foramen ovale

b.   Secundum atrial septal defect

c.   Partial anomalous pulmonary venous return

d.   Persistent left SVC

e.   Perimembranous ventricular septal defect

Atrial Septal Defect

If unrepaired, a large atrial septal defect may lead to pulmonary artery hypertension and atrial arrhythmias. There are four types of atrial septal defects: primum, secundum, PFO, and sinus venosus.

12.1   *Primum atrial septal defect* occurs close to the atrioventricular valves (Figures 12.1a and 12.1b) and shunts blood left to right. It is commonly associated with a *cleft anterior mitral leaflet* (Figure 12.1c) and is a common feature of Down syndrome.

> **LEARNING DIRECTIVE**
>
> **See Clip 12.2:** A short axis view shows the anterior mitral leaflet is cleft. Septal flattening is present as the result of RV volume/pressure overload.

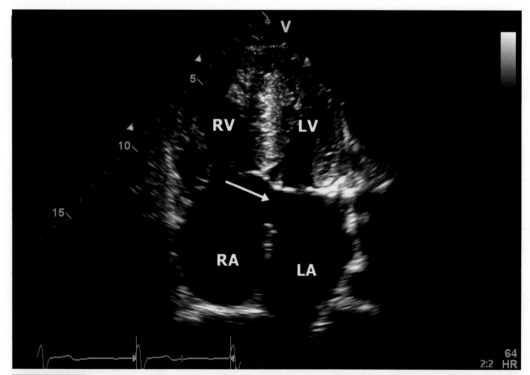

Figure 12.1a   TTE four-chamber view demonstrates a large primum ASD (arrow).

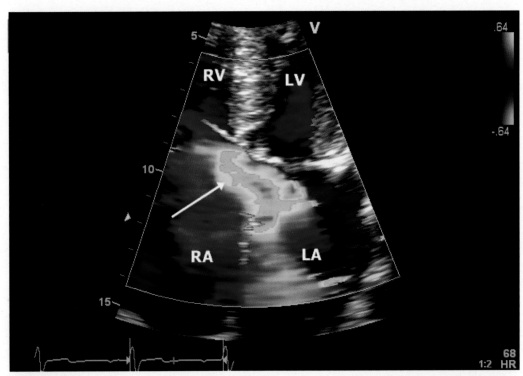

Figure 12.1b TTE four-chamber view demonstrates color Doppler flow across the defect (arrow).

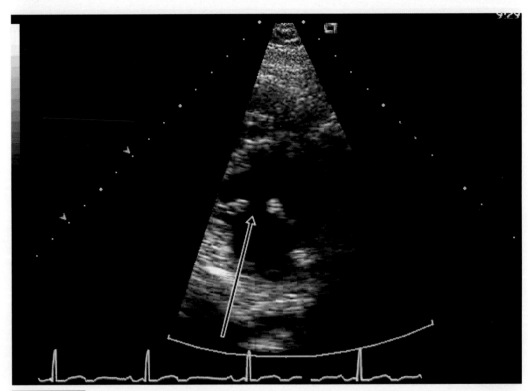

Figure 12.1c TTE parasternal short axis view of a cleft mitral leaflet (arrow). The patient also had a primum atrial septal defect.

The most extreme cases present as *common atrioventricular canal* with extension of the defect into the interventricular septum and a common atrioventricular valve (Figure 12.2).

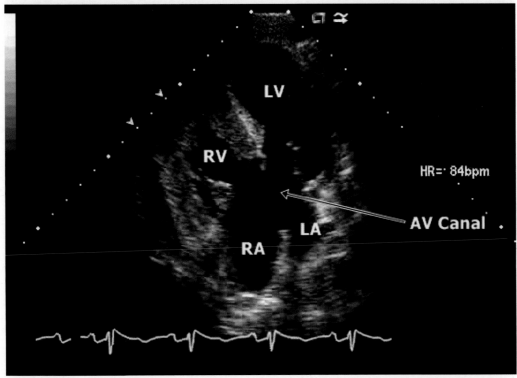

Figure 12.2 TTE apical four-chamber view demonstrating a common atrioventricular canal.

12.2 A *secundum atrial septal defect* is by far the most common atrial septal defect. The shunt is usually left-to-right (Figure 12.3). Secundum atrial septal defect may occur in isolation or in conjunction with an *atrial septal aneurysm*. Secundum atrial septal defect may be associated with mitral valve prolapse and is a common finding in *Ebstein Anomaly.*

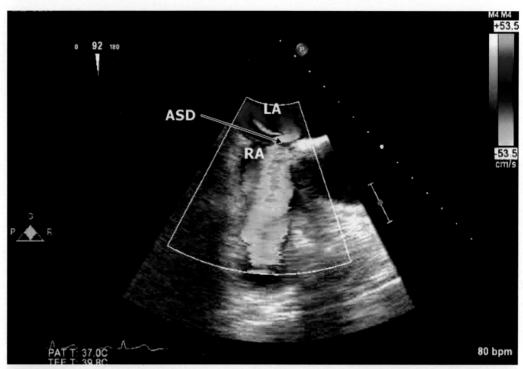

Figure 12.3   TEE in the midesophageal view at 90° demonstrates a large secundum atrial septal defect.

A common technique for identification of interatrial shunting is to inject agitated saline into the venous circulation. The bubbles present within the saline opacify the RA and will enter the LA through the shunt whenever RA pressure exceeds LA pressure. A persistent left-to-right shunt may produce a *negative contrast effect*, in which the flow through the atrial septal defect clears the contrast in the RA in a pulsatile fashion as it flows through the defect (see Figure 1.6).

12.3   *Patent foramen ovale (PFO)* occurs in up to one-third of patients, as documented by autopsy studies. Most PFOs are benign, but there is a troublesome and complex association between PFO and cryptogenic stroke, especially in younger patients. The value of TTE for detection of a cardiac source of embolism depends greatly upon concomitant evidence of cardiovascular disease. In the absence of any such findings, including normal sinus rhythm, a normal physical exam, and a normal electrocardiogram, the yield of TTE for PFO approaches 20%. By contrast, TEE produces a significant diagnostic yield for cardiac source of embolism even in the absence of other findings. Agitated saline plays an essential role in making the diagnosis in many patients (Figure 12.4a). Other clinical scenarios where identification of PFO has clinical relevance include hypoxia in the setting of an acute inferior wall myocardial infarction and pulmonary embolism, where elevated right heart pressures may produce transient right-to-left shunting and hypoxia through the defect. The number of bubbles passed relates roughly to the size of the PFO, with more than 30 bubbles suggesting a PFO size of greater than 4 mm. Echocardiography can also be used to guide the placement and evaluate the efficacy of percutaneous closure of the interatrial septum (Figures 12.4a–12.4c).

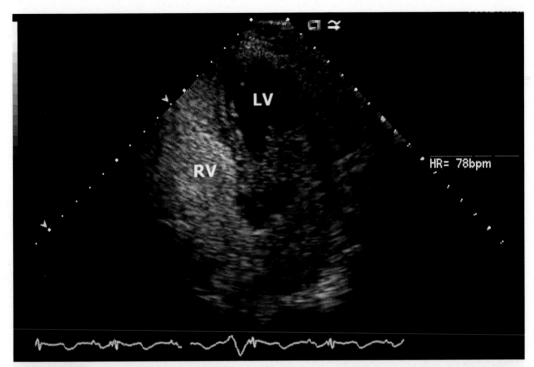

Figure 12.4a TTE in the four-chamber view with a markedly positive bubble study with bubbles in the LA and LV suggesting a large intracardiac shunt.

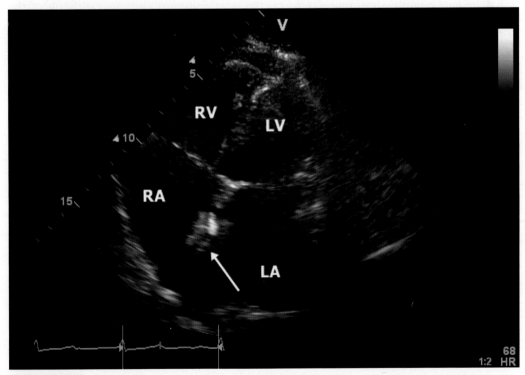

Figure 12.4b TTE four-chamber view in a patient with a properly placed intra-atrial septal closure device (arrow).

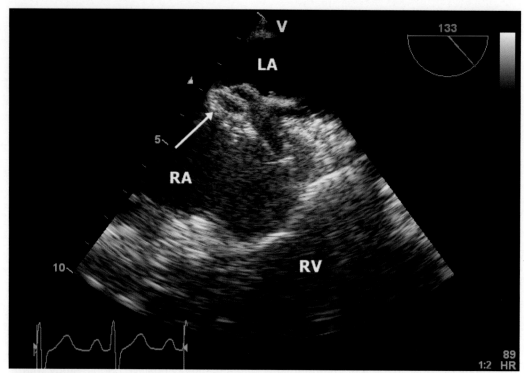

Figure 12.4c   TEE midesophageal view of an intra-atrial septal closure device (arrow).

12.4   *Sinus venosus atrial septal defect* is the least common and most difficult of the atrial septal defects to locate. In many cases, it is best seen by TEE in the bicaval view (Figure 12.5). Sinus venosus atrial septal defect is commonly associated with *anomalous pulmonary venous drainage*, most commonly of the right upper pulmonary vein.

LEARNING DIRECTIVE

See Clip 12.9: Anomalous pulmonary venous drainage into the RA at the superior vena cava–RA junction in this bicaval transesophageal view.

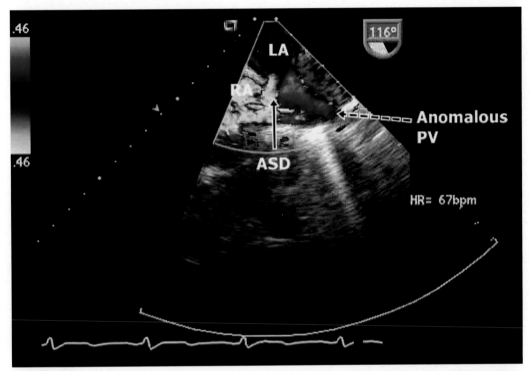

Figure 12.5 TEE bicaval view demonstrating a sinus venosus atrial septal defect (ASD, solid arrow) with associated partial anomalous pulmonary venous drainage.

Hemodynamically significant atrial septal defects produce RV volume overload as the result of excess flow into the RA. Typical signs include RV dilation, diastolic flattening (volume overload) of the interventricular septum, and paradoxical septal motion (pressure overload).

Ventricular Septal Defect

There are four types of ventricular septal defect: perimembranous, muscular, inlet, and supracristal.

12.5 *Perimembranous (also called subaortic) ventricular septal defect* is the most common in adults and is often seen on TTE in the parasternal long axis view as a flow from the LV just below the aortic root into the RV; in the parasternal short axis view, it is seen just below the level of the great vessels (Figure 12.6a). In the apical four-chamber view, the defect is seen just below the atrioventricular valves (Figure 12.6b).

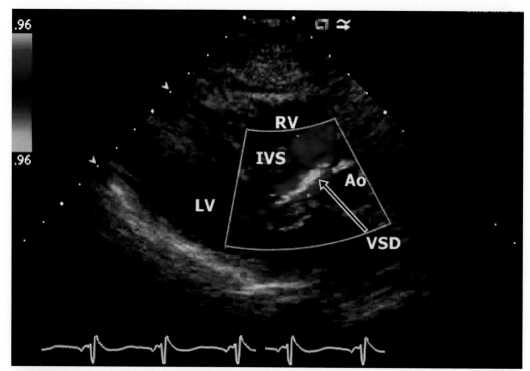

Figure 12.6a TTE parasternal long axis view demonstrating a perimembranous (subaortic) ventricular septal defect (VSD). Note the subaortic location of left-to-right-flow on color Doppler.

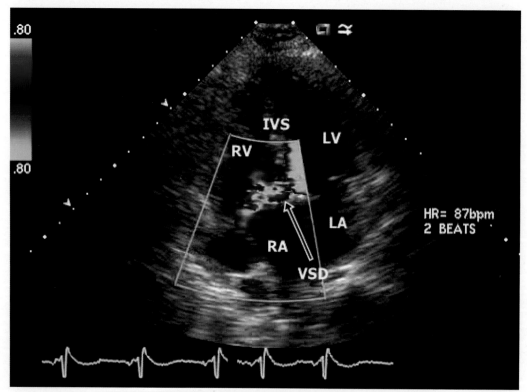

Figure 12.6b TTE apical four-chamber view demonstrating a perimembranous ventricular septal defect (VSD), with left-to-right flow seen on color Doppler originating in the LVOT just below the aortic valve (arrow).

Perimembranous ventricular septal defects comprise the majority of ventricular septal defects, with a frequency approaching 80% of all such defects. The defect commonly closes in childhood.

12.6 *Muscular ventricular septal defects* are the most common defects in newborns. Most close spontaneously as the child ages. The defects are often located toward the apex and may be multiple (Figure 12.7). Size may vary greatly. "Pinhole" defects are clinically inconsequential and often close spontaneously, but larger defects may persist and lead to heart failure.

> **LEARNING DIRECTIVE**
>
> **See Clip 12.23:** Left-to-right flow across the defect.

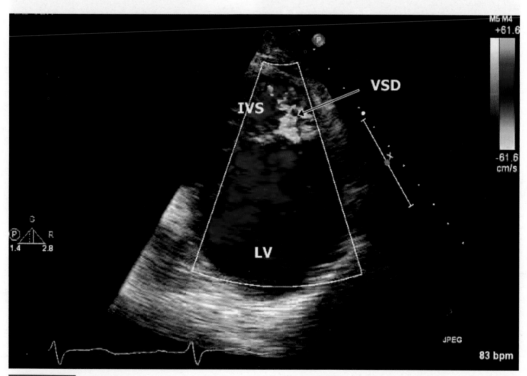

Figure 12.7 TTE from parasternal short axis view demonstrating a muscular ventricular septal defect (arrow).

12.7 *Inlet ventricular septal defect* is usually seen in a four-chamber view as a defect close to the insertion of the septal tricuspid leaflet (Figure 12.8). Cleft mitral valve may also be seen.

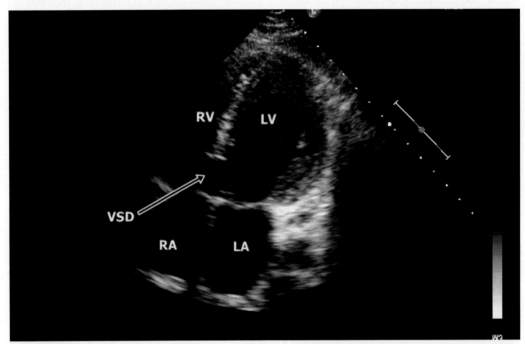

Figure 12.8 TTE in the apical four-chamber view demonstrating an inlet ventricular septal defect (VSD).

12.8 *Supracristal (or "subpulmonic" because of its location) ventricular septal defect* is the least common of the ventricular septal defects. It involves the outlet septum just below the pulmonic valve (Figures 12.9a).

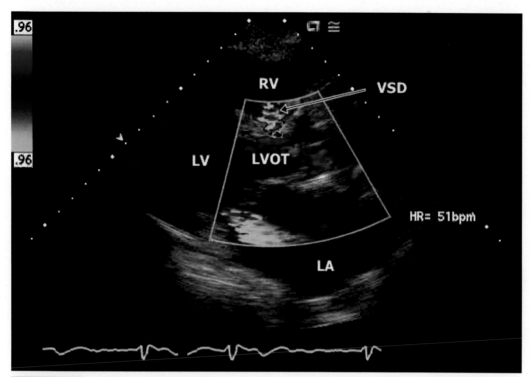

Figure 12.9a TTE in the parasternal long axis demonstrates a supracristal ventricular septal defect. In this view, the defect appears similar to perimembranous ventricular septal defect.

Supracristal ventricular septal defect can be challenging to differentiate from perimembranous ventricular septal defect because both defects are seen in a similar location in the parasternal long axis view, but a high-parasternal short axis view will distinguish between the two. Supracristal ventricular septal defect flow will be seen at about 1 o'clock from just below the aortic valve into the RVOT (Figure 12.9b), while perimembranous ventricular septal defect flow will be seen at approximately 10 o'clock. A supracristal defect is commonly associated with aortic regurgitation as the result of aortic leaflet prolapse. An apical five-chamber view will show flow from LVOT into the RV.

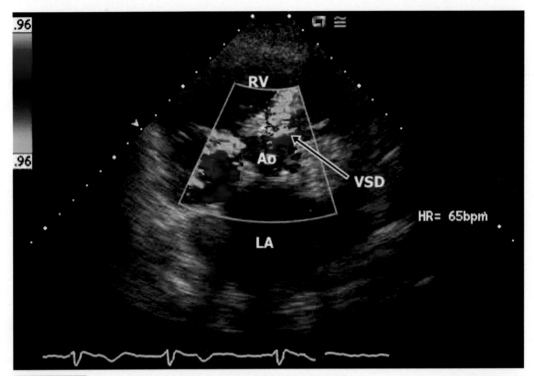

Figure 12.9b   A parasternal short axis view of a supracristal ventricular septal defect (VSD) shows flow below the aorta (arrow).

12.9   *Calculating the magnitude of left-to-right shunt*: To calculate the Q_p/Q_s, or ratio of pulmonary to systemic flow, simply calculate the RV stroke volume and divide by the LV stroke volume:

$$\frac{(0.785)(D_{RVOT})^2(VTI_{RVOT})}{(0.785)(D_{LVOT})^2(VTI_{LVOT})}$$

Note the equation simplifies nicely to:

$$\frac{(D_{RVOT})^2(VTI_{RVOT})}{(D_{LVOT})^2(VTI_{LVOT})}$$

Therefore, if $D_{RVOT} = 1.8$ cm, $VTI_{RVOT} = 40$ cm, $D_{LVOT} = 2$ cm, and $VTI_{LVOT} = 25$ cm, then the formula solves as:

$$Q_p/Q_s = \frac{(1.8^2)(40)}{(2^2)(25)} = 1.3:1$$

12.10 *Eisenmenger syndrome* is the most feared complication of a large ventricular septal defect. In this syndrome, increased pulmonary flow eventually leads to obliteration of the normal pulmonary vasculature with resultant pulmonary hypertension and reversal of the shunt from left-to-right to right-to-left. RV dilation and dysfunction will inevitably be present. Echocardiographic findings include pulmonary artery dilatation, RV free wall hypertrophy, tricuspid regurgitation, and flattening of the interventricular septum throughout the cardiac cycle. In this stage, bidirectional flow through the defect may be seen by color Doppler flow interrogation.

12.11 *Coarctation of the aorta*: Aortic coarctations most commonly occur distal to the ligamentum arteriosum just beyond the subclavian artery (Figure 12.10). In a majority of cases, a *bicuspid aortic valve* is also present. Coarctation is best seen in the suprasternal view. The gradient across the coarctation can be interrogated by both color-flow and spectral Doppler.

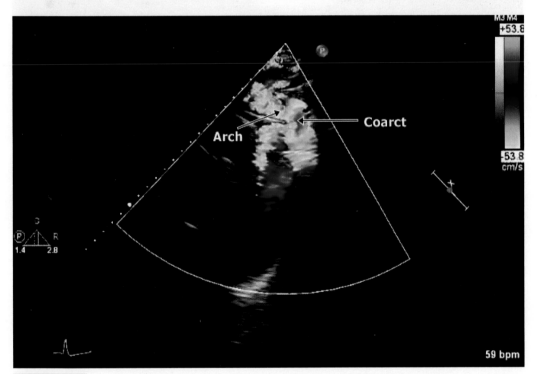

Figure 12.10 TTE suprasternal view demonstrating coarctation of the aorta.

12.12 *Bicuspid aortic valve* is the most common adult congenital anomaly. It usually presents with a fish-mouth appearance and a residual raphe representing the missing cusp. The defect is best seen in the parasternal short axis view. The most common configuration for the valve is to open 9 o'clock to 3 o'clock, but it can appear in any form. Both aortic stenosis and regurgitation are common, and bicuspid aortic valve is the most common cause of aortic stenosis in middle age. The parasternal long axis view will often demonstrate systolic doming and an eccentric closure point (Figure 12.11).

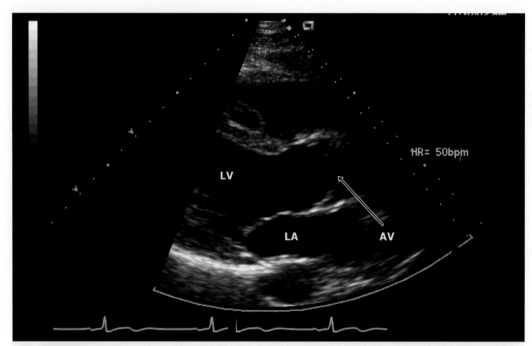

Figure 12.11   TTE parasternal long axis view demonstrating a bicuspid aortic valve (AV) with systolic doming.

12.13 *Pulmonic stenosis* can be infundibular (as in tetralogy of Fallot) or valvular. Pulmonic stenosis is often challenging to image well in adults. The diagnosis depends upon determining an accurate gradient across the pulmonic valve in the short axis view. An M-mode showing the classic "W" sign (see Figures 9.7–9.9) may be helpful, and the spectral Doppler pattern will show acceleration of flow with a steep upslope as discussed previously.

12.14 *Patent ductus arteriosus*: A patent ductus arteriosus is best seen from either the high-left parasternal view (Figure 12.12a) or a parasternal short axis view at the aortic/pulmonary artery level (Figure 12.12b).

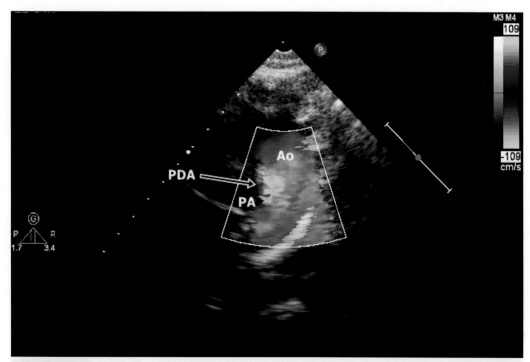

Figure 12.12a TTE suprasternal view demonstrating flow from the distal aortic arch into the pulmonary artery (PA) through a patent ductus arteriosus (PDA) as seen in the "ductal view."

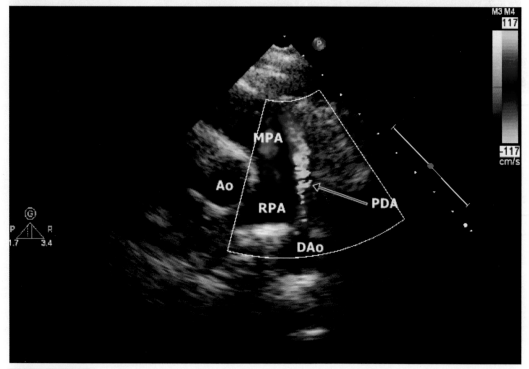

Figure 12.12b TTE parasternal short axis view demonstrating flow from the patent ductus arteriosus (PDA) emerging from the descending aorta (DAo) into the main pulmonary artery (MPA).

Flow in either view can be seen from the aorta into the left pulmonary artery at its takeoff from the main pulmonary artery. Patent ductus arteriosus is most commonly an isolated lesion. If the shunt is large enough, *diastolic flow reversal* may be seen in the descending aorta. Pulmonary artery systolic pressure may be calculated by subtracting the patent ductus arteriousus gradient from the systolic blood pressure.

12.15 *Tetrology of Fallot* (Figure 12.13) is a complex and often cyanotic lesion composed of RV hypertrophy, infundibular pulmonic stenosis, a nonrestrictive ventricular septal defect, and an overriding aorta.

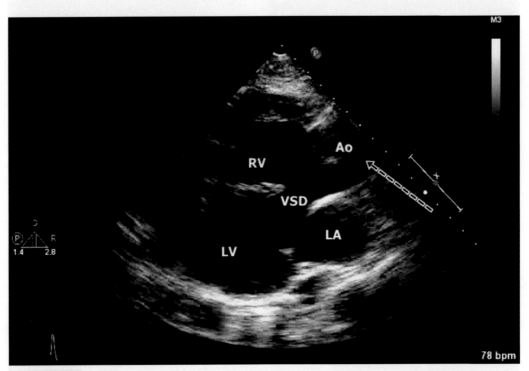

Figure 12.13   TTE parasternal long axis view demonstrating tetrology of Fallot, with a large nonrestrictive ventricular septal defect (VSD) and overriding aorta (arrow).

LEARNING DIRECTIVE

See Clip 12.39: The VSD demonstrates a large left-to-right shunt by color flow.

12.16 The anomaly produces several echocardiographic hallmarks, most of which are seen in the parasternal long axis and apical four-chamber views. Other defects, including an atrial septal defect, a right aortic arch, and pulmonary artery hypoplasia, are commonly seen. Initial palliative measures for tetrology have included systemic-to-pulmonary shunts to allow blood to bypass the pulmonary artery obstruction and accept oxygen. Examples include the *Blalock-Taussig shunt* (subclavian to pulmonary artery), *Waterston shunt* (ascending aorta to right pulmonary artery), and *Potts shunt* (descending aorta to left pulmonary artery). In the current era, primary complete surgical correction is provided in early childhood whenever possible.

12.17 *Truncus arteriosus* is a morphologic cousin of tetrology of Fallot but differs critically from it by the presence of a single outlet arising from both the RV and LV. The single truncal root then gives rise to both the aorta and the pulmonary artery. In a truncus, the conotruncal anatomy can best be seen in a high-parasternal short axis view.

12.18 When the great arteries are switched, the condition is known as *d-transposition* (for normal dextro- or rightward looping of the embryologic ventricles). The ventricles are in the right place, but the RV is connected directly to the aorta and the LV is connected to the pulmonary artery. This disease is uniformly fatal unless another communication between left and right heart is also present, because the right and left heart circuits function in parallel. An atrial septal defect is frequently present, or is created after delivery by an *atrial septostomy* (Rashkind procedure), which allows mixing of oxygenated and unoxygenated blood. Before the arterial switch procedure became readily available (late 1980s), palliation was provided via the *Mustard* or *Senning* procedures, in which an atrial baffle redirects blood from the RA into the LV, and from the LA into the RV (Figure 12.14a). The procedure allows oxygenated blood to reach the systemic circulation but does not solve the long-term problems of using the RV as a systemic ventricle. A common complication of the procedure is stenosis of the superior vena caval limb of the systemic venous baffle (Figure 12.14b). In the short axis view at the level of the ventricles, the systemic RV is hypertrophied and the septum bows into the thin-walled LV.

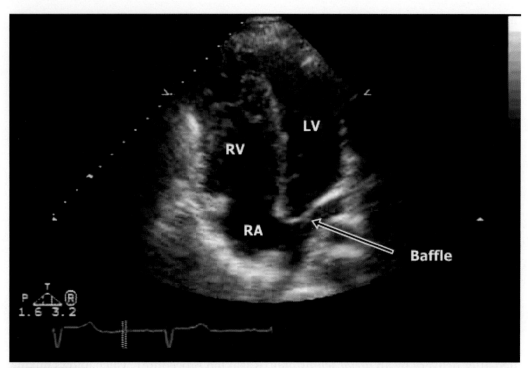

Figure 12.14a   TTE apical four-chamber view demonstrating d-transposition of the great arteries with an atrial baffle (arrow) in place.

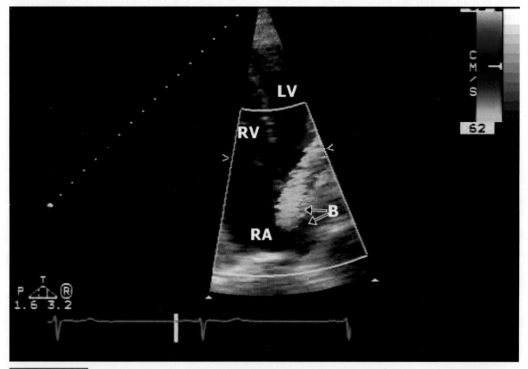

Figure 12.14b   TTE in the apical four-chamber view demonstrating high-velocity flow through the atrial baffle from the superior vena cava inlet indicating baffle (B) stenosis.

12.19 If both the great arteries and the ventricles are switched, the condition is called *l-transposition* (for levorotation of the embryologic ventricles). Alternative names include *congenitally corrected transposition* and *ventricular inversion*. In this circumstance, the unoxygenated blood from the RA enters the morphologic LV (on the right side), flows into the pulmonary artery, returns to the LA via the pulmonary veins, enters the morphologic RV (on the left side), and exits the aorta. The normal circulation in the series is maintained and there is no cyanosis, but the morphologic RV and LV have switched positions, with the RV functioning as the systemic ventricle. Embryologically, this is a very different condition than d-transposition; its genesis begins with abnormal embryologic looping of the ventricles versus abnormal rotation of the aorta and pulmonary artery. Common associated features include ventricular septal defect, pulmonary stenosis, regurgitation of the systemic tricuspid valve, and heart block (Figure 12.15).

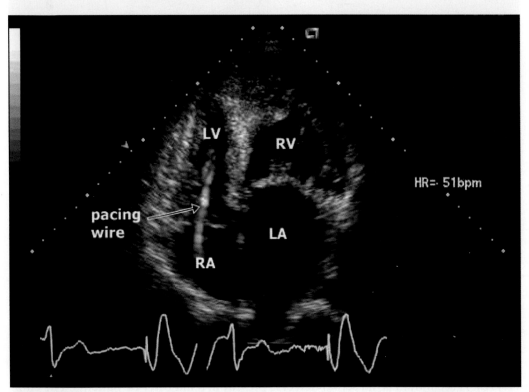

Figure 12.15 TTE in the apical four-chamber view demonstrates l-transposition. A pacemaker lead was placed in the morphologic LV for high-degree atrioventricular block.

In both forms of transposition, the great vessels are *parallel to each other at their origin*. In the short axis view, both the aorta and the pulmonary artery are seen in cross section, the aorta displaced superiorly and to the left in l-transposition and superiorly to the right in d-transposition (Figure 12.16).

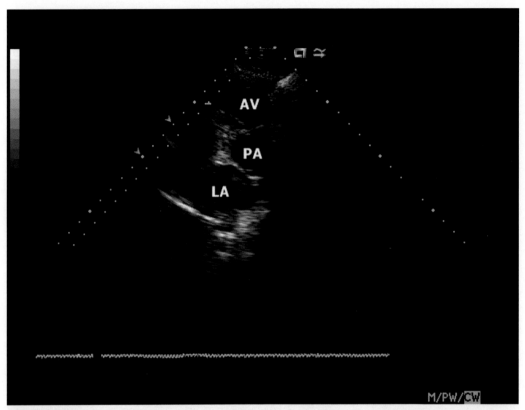

Figure 12.16   Parasternal short axis view of d-transposition demonstrating the great vessels in parallel. The aorta is displaced anterior and to the right of the pulmonic artery (PA).

The diagnosis of l-transposition can be made from the apical four-chamber view alone, since the morphologic RV and the tricuspid valve are now located on the patient's left side. The apical displacement of the tricuspid valve (which is always part of the morphologic RV) is a key feature in the RV's location. Other features include a moderator band (if visible) and RV trabeculation.

12.20 *Ebstein anomaly* is a complex condition characterized by an apically displaced tricuspid valve with a "sail" septal leaflet and ventricularized RA (Figures 12.17a and 12.17b). A secundum atrial septal defect is present in a majority of patients. The clinical presentation is highly variable and can range from intermittent cyanosis to asymptomatic. The apically displaced tricuspid valve is demonstrated in both the parasternal short axis and the apical four-chamber views.

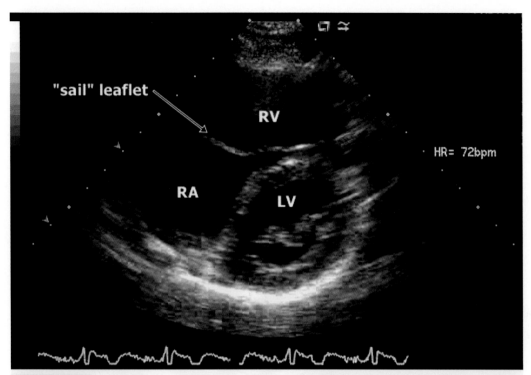

Figure 12.17a   TTE in the parasternal short axis view in a patient with Ebstein anomaly. The large sail-like septal leaflet of the tricuspid valve (arrow) is displaced anteriorly, and signs of pulmonary hypertension are present, with RV enlargement and systolic flattening of the interventricular septum.

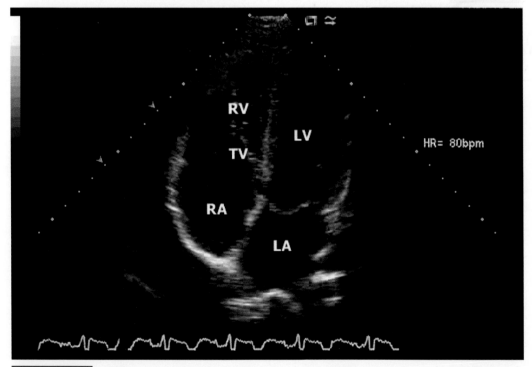

Figure 12.17b   TTE in the apical four-chamber view from the same patient showing typical features of Ebstein anomaly. Note the apically displaced insertion of the septal leaflet of the tricuspid valve (TV).

12.21 *Tricuspid atresia* is a complex and always cyanotic defect producing an atretic tricuspid valve and an often small, nonfunctioning RV (Figure 12.18).

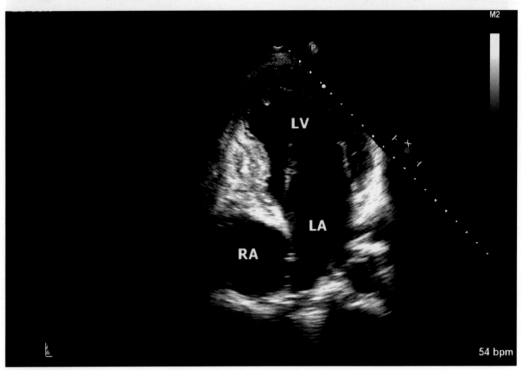

Figure 12.18   TEE in the apical four-chamber view in a patient with tricuspid atresia. Note absence of a functioning tricuspid valve and RV.

Desaturated blood is shunted directly past the lungs into the left side via an atrial septal defect. As an echocardiographer of adult patients, you will likely never see this disease without some sort of palliation. The most common early palliation is a systemic to pulmonary shunt to relieve cyanosis. The original version, the *Blalock-Taussig shunt*, which connected the left subclavian artery to the pulmonary artery, has largely been replaced by the *bidirectional Glenn shunt*, which connects the superior vena cava to the pulmonary artery. Definitive palliation is provided by the *Fontan* operation (Figure 12.19), which bypasses the right heart by creating a pass-through from the inferior vena cava and the superior vena cava directly into the pulmonary artery. This same operation can be used for *hypoplastic left heart syndrome* or any other form of single-ventricle defect.

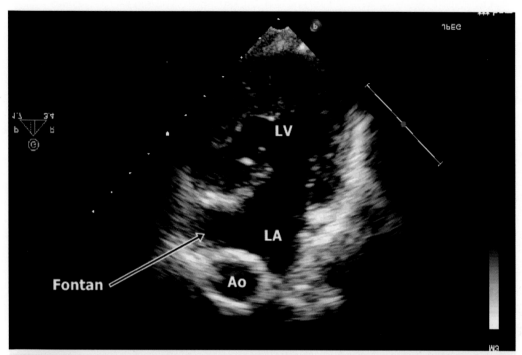

Figure 12.19 TTE in the apical four-chamber view in a patient who has undergone a Fontan procedure (arrow) due to tricuspid atresia.

12.22 *Cor triatriatum* is among the rarest of congenital anomalies (Figures 12.20a and 12.20b). It occurs when a membrane is produced by a failure of complete reabsorption between the embryologic common pulmonary veins to the back of the LA. The membrane may obstruct pulmonary venous return to produce pseudomitral stenosis or may produce no hemodynamic abnormalities. The membrane is curved, may have a wind-sock contour, and moves toward the mitral valve plane in diastole. All pulmonary veins drain proximal to the membrane. The LA appendage and foramen ovale are located on the "LV side" of the membrane. An atrial septal defect, either proximal or distal to the membrane, is often present. In contrast, a *supramitral ring* attaches to the base of the mitral valve past the LA appendage and foramen ovale. In this condition, obstruction of mitral inflow may produce mitral stenosis.

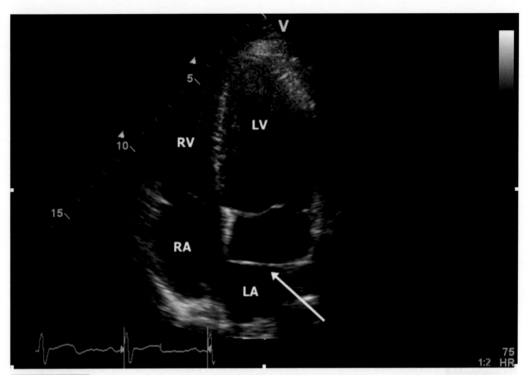

Figure 12.20a   TTE four-chamber view demonstrates cor triatriatum in the LA (arrow).

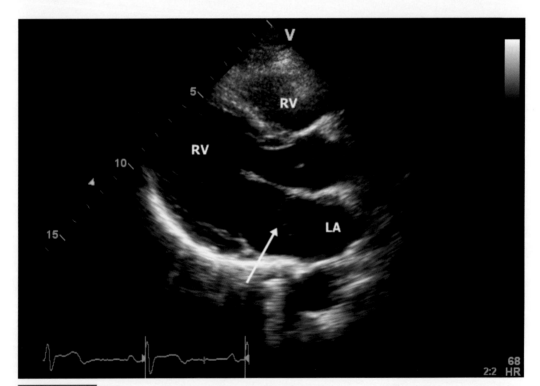

Figure 12.20b   TTE parasternal long axis view demonstrates cor triatriatum.

12.23 *Dilated coronary sinus/persistent left superior vena cava* is a common normal variant in which the left superior vena cava is not reabsorbed and empties directly into a *dilated coronary sinus*. The dilated coronary sinus can usually be seen tucked just behind the posterior mitral valve leaflet in parasternal long axis view (Figure 12.21). The anomaly is confirmed by injection of agitated saline into the left brachial vein, with appearance of agitated saline in the coronary sinus followed by the RA.

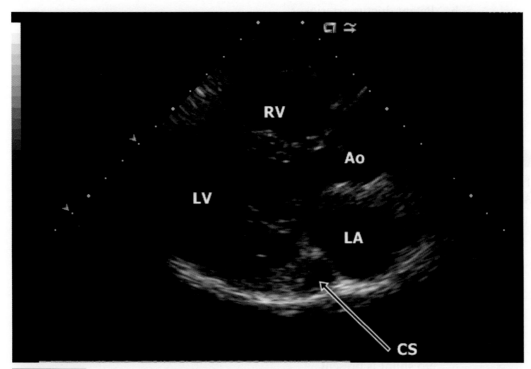

Figure 12.21   TTE parasternal long axis view demonstrates a dilated coronary sinus (CS) in a patient with persistent left superior vena cava. Other less common causes of a dilated coronary sinus include coronary artery to coronary sinus fistula, anomalous pulmonary venous drainage, and an unroofed atrial septal defect emptying into the coronary sinus.

ADVANCED QUESTIONS

Q12.4 Which of the following congenital heart disease conditions produces holo-diastolic flow reversal in the descending aorta?

a. Congenital aortic stenosis

b. Patent ductus arteriosus

c. Perimembranous ventricular septal defect

d. Ebstein anomaly

e. L-transposition

Q12.5 Injection of the left antecubital fossa with agitated saline produces the appearance of bubbles within the LA six cardiac cycles after their appearance within the RA. The location of the shunt is?

a. Interatrial

b. Interventricular

c. Intrapulmonary

d. Intraarterial

e. No shunt is present.

Q12.6 During injection of agitated saline, an atrial septal defect will often produce a negative contrast effect. Which flow can mimic this effect and produce a false-positive study?

a. High-volume superior vena caval flow

b. High-volume inferior vena caval flow

c. Tricuspid regurgitation

d. Tricuspid stenosis

e. Partial anomalous pulmonary venous return

Q12.7 Which congenital anomaly is not well seen from the four-chamber view?

    a. Muscular ventricular septal defect

    b. Ebstein anomaly

    c. Inlet ventricular septal defect

    d. L-transposition

    e. Perimembranous (subaortic) ventricular septal defect

Q12.8 Which congenital anomaly most commonly produces aortic regurgitation as a direct hemodynamic consequence?

    a. Supracristal ventricular septal defect

    b. Muscular ventricular septal defect

    c. Primum atrial septal defect

    d. Perimembranous (subaortic) ventricular septal defect

    e. Ebstein's anomaly

Q12.9 Which echocardiographic view distinguishes truncus arteriosus from tetrology of Fallot?

    a. Parasternal long axis

    b. Parasternal short axis

    c. Apical four-chamber

    d. Apical two-chamber

    e. Apical three-chamber

Q12.10 A persistent left superior vena cava is most commonly associated with which of the following findings?

    a. Partial anomalous pulmonary venous drainage

    b. Atrial septal aneurysm

    c. Dilated coronary sinus

    d. Atrial septal aneurysm

    e. Cor triatriatum

Q12.11 The anatomic RV can be determined by the:

    a. Size of the chamber

    b. Connection to the pulmonary artery

    c. Connection to the tricuspid valve

    d. Thickness of the free wall

    e. Connection to the superior vena cava

Q12.12 A patient with persistent left superior vena cava is injected with agitated saline through the right brachial vein. Where does the contrast effect produced by the saline first appear?

    a. RA

    b. RV

    c. LA

    d. LV

    e. Coronary sinus

Q12.13 The patient with the congenital anomaly shown in Figure Q12.13 will often present with:

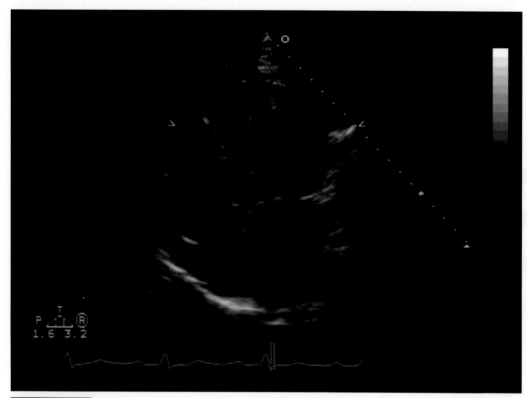

Figure Q12.13

a. No symptoms

b. Vasovagal syncope

c. Chest pain

d. Variable cyanosis

e. Pulmonary hypertension

For Questions 12.14–12.16, match the operation with the congenital heart defect.

    a.   Hypopolastic left heart syndrome or tricuspid atresia

    b.   Tetrology of Fallot

    c.   Atrial septal defect

    d.   Bicuspid aortic valve

    e.   D-transposition of the great vessels

Q12.14   Fontan

Q12.15   Blalock-Taussig

Q12.16   Mustard, Senning, or arterial switch

ANSWERS

Q12.4   b: Runoff from the aorta to the pulmonary artery produces holodiastolic flow reversal. Other conditions exhibiting this phenomenon include aortic regurgitation and systemic-to-pulmonary shunts such as the Blalock-Taussig. (Section **12.16**)

Q12.5   c: Intrapulmonary shunts produce a delayed appearance of contrast material in the LA. (Section **1.23**)

Q12.6   b: See Section **1.23**.

Q12.7   e: Perimembranous (subaortic) ventricular septal defect is best seen in views that show the LVOT. The other four choices are well seen in an apical four-chamber view. (Section **12.5**)

Q12.8   d: Perimembranous ventricular septal defect produces aortic regurgitation via the Venturi effect and in so doing increases the risk of endocarditis. (Section **12.5**)

Q12.9   b: The parasternal short axis will demonstrate the presence of a single outflow valve in truncus arteriosus. In the parasternal long axis view, the two conditions may be indistinguishable. (Sections **12.16** and **12.17**)

Q12.10   c: See Section **12.23**.

Q12.11   c: The tricuspid valve, which lies closer to the apex than the mitral valve, establishes the location of the morphologic RV. (Section **12.18**)

Q12.12   a: This is a trick question. Patients with a persistent left superior vena cava also have a normal superior vena cava in the proper location. (Section **12.23**)

Q12.13   a: This is congenitally corrected or l-transposition. Note the position of the anatomic RV. The presence of a pacemaker notwithstanding, many patients may be asymptomatic early in life until the pressure load imposed upon the systemic RV takes its toll. (Section **12.18**)

Q12.14   a: See Section **12.21**.

Q12.15   b: See Section **12.15**.

Q12.16   e: See Section **12.18**.

13

TAMPONADE, CONSTRICTION, AND RESTRICTION

PRACTICE QUESTIONS

For Questions 13.1–13.4, match the respiratory change with the variable.

    a.   Increases with inspiration

    b.   Increases with expiration

    c.   Does not change with respiration

Q13.1   Degree of tricuspid regurgitation in an otherwise normal patient

Q13.2   Isovolumic relaxation time in a patient with constrictive pericarditis

Q13.3   Peak transmitral inflow (E wave) in a patient with restrictive physiology

Q13.4   Peak transmitral inflow velocity in a patient with cardiac tamponade

ANSWERS: 13.1. a; 13.2. a; 13.3. c; 13.4. b

13.1   Tamponade, myocardial restriction, and pericardial constriction all produce reduced filling on both sides of the heart, but the cause is different in each case. In constriction, a rigid external barrier limits inflow. Think of an otherwise normal heart that cannot expand because it is placed inside of a box. Because both ventricles are encased in the same barrier, they are now interconnected, a phenomenon known as *ventricular interdependence*. The external impediment to filling means that the only portion of the heart that moves in diastole is the interventricular septum. When blood enters one side, it is excluded from the other side and the septum shifts toward the less filled side. Also described as "septal shift and shudder," this sign, when present, can be appreciated by M-mode echocardiography at the level of the LV (Figure 13.1).

> **LEARNING DIRECTIVE**
>
> **See Clip 13.15:** Note the septal "shift and shudder" in this patient with constriction.

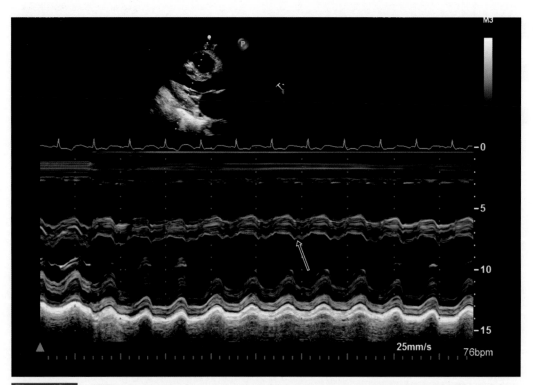

Figure 13.1   TTE parasternal long axis view. M-mode demonstrates septal "shift and shudder," or septal notching (arrow), typical of constrictive pericarditis.

Consequently, respiration produces the opposite effect from one side of the heart to the next. With inspiration, right-sided blood flow increases, the septum pushes into the left side, left-sided filling falls, and *isovolumic relaxation time increases* as the decrease in left-sided filling prolongs the time to mitral valve opening. Thus, the diastolic component of pulmonary vein inflow (PV_d) decreases with inspiration. With expiration, the sequence reverses: IVRT decreases, PV_d increases, right-sided filling decreases, and the normal diastolic forward flow from the hepatic vein is reversed (Figure 13.2).

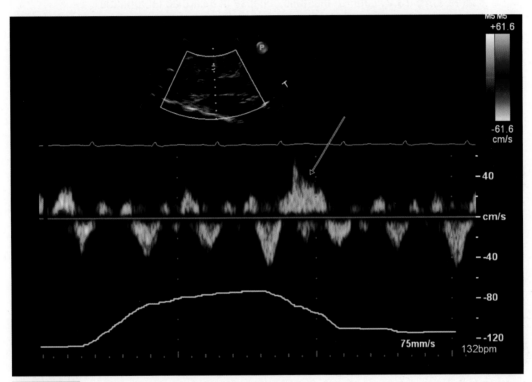

Figure 13.2 TTE in the subcostal view demonstrates hepatic vein flow reversal (arrow) during expiration. The bottom line tracks respiration.

13.2 The hemodynamic definition of cardiac tamponade is met when the fluid-filled pericardial space causes intrapericardial pressure to rise above RV end-diastolic pressure. This reversal of the normal relationship between intrapericardial pressure and right-sided diastolic pressure restricts right-sided inflow and produces a characteristic set of echocardiographic findings. In rough order of increasing specificity, they include:

1. *Effusion.* A pericardial effusion does not need to be large to cause hemodynamic compromise. The development of tamponade depends upon the rate of accumulation. Partial or loculated effusion or a thrombus behind the RA or RV can also produce tamponade physiology, most commonly after cardiac surgery or chest trauma.

2. *Late diastolic collapse of the RA.* The low-pressure RA is most sensitive to the increase in intrapericardial pressure. Diastolic LA collapse can also be seen in up to 30% of cases. RA collapse is a highly sensitive sign for tamponade (Figure 13.3a).

LEARNING DIRECTIVE

See Clip 13.2: Late RA diastolic collapse in a cardiac tamponade.

3. *Early diastolic RV collapse.* The normal rapid rise in RV diastolic pressure is blunted by the resistance to further expansion from the fluid-filled intrapericardial space. This sign is specific for tamponade (Figure 13.3b).

4. *Marked septal respiratory variation.* The leftward shift of the septum with inspiration decreases left-sided stroke volume and produces a transient decline in systolic pressure, producing the pulses paradoxus.

5. *Swinging heart sign.*

LEARNING DIRECTIVE

See Clip 13.7: Swinging heart sign in the four-chamber view.

6. *Respiratory variation of mitral inflow.* A decrease of greater than 25% in peak transmitral E wave during inspiration is a highly useful sign for tamponade (Figure 13.4). Respiration has the opposite effect on the right side. Tricuspid inflow demonstrates an exaggeration of the normal increase with inspiration and decrease with expiration. On the left side, a respirometer is not required for recognition of this sign, since the normal pattern is that the left side is insensitive to respiratory variation.

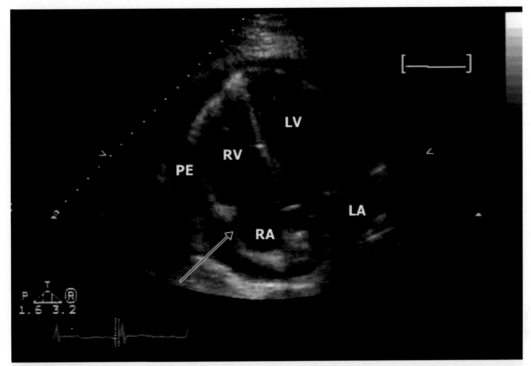

Figure 13.3a TTE in the parasternal four-chamber view demonstrates diastolic RA collapse (arrow) in this patient with atrial fibrillation and pericardial effusion (PE).

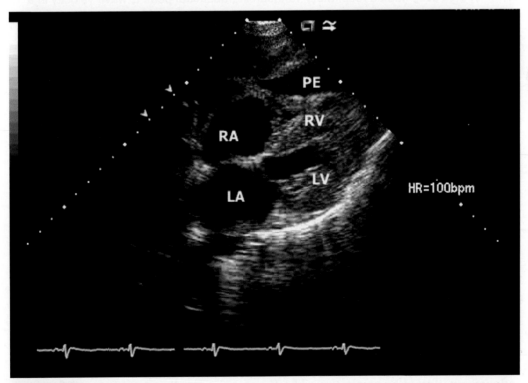

Figure 13.3b TTE in the subcostal view in a patient with a moderate pericardial effusion (PE). Note the early diastolic collapse of the RV.

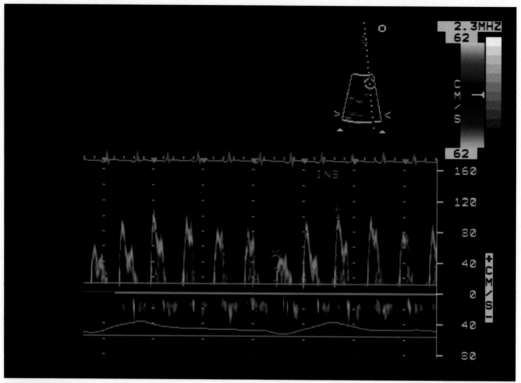

Figure 13.4 TTE in the four-chamber view. Respiratory inflow across the mitral valve demonstrates accentuated respiratory variation in transmitral peak E wave velocity in a patient with tamponade.

Right-sided findings of tamponade may be attenuated in the presence of pulmonary hypertension as the elevated pulmonary artery pressure acts as hemodynamic counterweight against the elevated intrapericardial pressure.

Restrictive Physiology

13.3 In restriction, the barrier is internal. The high LA pressure created as a consequence of restriction produces a variety of signs that characterize the diagnosis, including loss of PV_s, widened PV_a, and pulmonary venous hypertension. Transmitral E wave velocity is high and deceleration time is short. E' is low because the myocardium does not relax. In tamponade and constriction, there is nothing wrong with the myocardium, so parameters of intrinsic relaxation such as E' are unaffected.

13.4 Respiration produces critical differences in several echocardiographic signs that can be used to distinguish restriction from constriction. In restriction, mitral inflow is unaffected by respiration. The Kussmaul sign (decreased forward flow with inspiration) is absent. Diastolic hepatic vein flow reverses with inspiration (the opposite of tamponade and constriction), and the IVRT is unaffected because filling is insensitive to respiration. There are no signs of ventricular interdependence. In pericardial constriction, the normal relationship between E/E′ and LV end-diastolic pressure is inverted. E/E′ falls as LV end-diastolic pressure rises because the normal longitudinal motion of the annulus is exaggerated as LV end-diastolic pressure increases.

ADVANCED QUESTIONS

Q13.5   A deceleration time of < 130 msec is most consistent with:

    a.   Pulmonary systolic hypertension

    b.   Normal diastolic function

    c.   Elevated left atrial pressure

    d.   Left-to-right shunt

    e.   Patient prosthetic mismatch

Q13.6   Which hemodynamic abnormality reduces the specificity of diastolic RV collapse for the diagnosis of tamponade?

    a.   Pulmonary hypertension

    b.   Severe tricuspid regurgitation

    c.   Systemic hypertension

    d.   Elevated central venous pressure

    e.   Atrial septal defect

Q13.7   Which echocardiographic finding is most sensitive for detection of cardiac tamponade?

    a.   Hepatic vein systolic flow reversal

    b.   Respiratory variation in transmitral inflow of $\geq 40\%$

    c.   Early diastolic RA collapse

    d.   Equalization of LA and RV diastolic pressure

    e.   Massive pericardial effusion

Q13.8 Which echocardiographic finding is commonly seen in restriction?

a. Inverse correlation between E/E′ and LV end-diastolic pressure

b. Pulmonary hypertension

c. Expiratory reversal of hepatic vein inflow in diastole

d. Kussmaul sign

e. Diastolic RA collapse

ANSWERS

Q13.5   c: Deceleration time depends entirely upon the atrioventricular gradient in diastole. When LA pressure is elevated, the time to equilibration between the two chambers, the deceleration time, is shortened. (Section **13.1**)

Q13.6   a: Elevated pulmonary artery systolic pressure can attenuate the classical right-sided findings of tamponade, including both RA diastolic and RV diastolic collapse. (Section **13.2**)

Q13.7   c: See Section **13.2**.

Q13.8   b: All the other signs listed are seen either in pericardial constriction or in cardiac tamponade. (Sections **13.2** and **13.4**)

14 ENDOCARDITIS AND PROSTHETIC VALVE EVALUATION

Q14.1 The tissue density of valvular vegetation in endocarditis most closely resembles:

a. Blood

b. Thrombus

c. Pericardial fluid

d. Calcium

e. Myocardium

Q14.2 You are asked by the infectious disease service to evaluate a patient for TEE. TTE is of excellent quality and reveals a 5-mm irregular echodense mass on the anterior mitral leaflet with concomitant moderate mitral regurgitation. LV systolic function is normal, and there are no other valvular abnormalities. The patient is febrile with documented *Streptococcus viridans* bacteremia from two consecutive blood cultures obtained one hour apart, but is otherwise clinically stable. You now recommend:

a. Immediate TEE

b. Follow-up TEE in one week

c. Routine follow-up TTE at the end of six weeks of antibiotic therapy

d. No further echocardiographic follow-up unless there is evidence of clinical deterioration

Q14.3 Which of the following echocardiographic variables is an important predictor of outcome in patients with endocarditis?

a. Vegetation location

b. Presence of regurgitation

c. Increase in size

d. Decrease in size

e. Multileaflet involvement

Endocarditis

14.1 Echocardiography is a critical tool for establishing the diagnosis of endocarditis and identifying a variety of complications that directly affect management. An echocardiogram provides two vital types of information: (1) It supports or refutes the diagnosis, and (2) it provides data about the integrity of valvular function, the presence or absence of complications, and the likelihood of successful resolution or infection with medical therapy alone. While echocardiographic criteria for endocarditis are qualitative, several common descriptors are nearly universal.

14.2 *The presence of concomitant valvular regurgitation.* While it is possible to have native valve endocarditis without regurgitation, such cases are distinctly uncommon. The pathogenesis of the disease depends upon regurgitation to produce the turbulence that leads to endothelial surface disruption and provides a nidus for bacterial adherence and consequent infection. The absence of any regurgitation should raise suspicions about the viability of the diagnosis.

14.3 *The characteristics of the suspected vegetation:* This is surely the toughest criterion. Ultrasound only provides information about the shape and relative brightness or echodensity of a structure, and echocardiographers then make inferences about the identity and characteristics of that structure based on accumulated experience. For vegetations, there is a continuum of echodensity, shape, size, and mobility along which the certainty of diagnosis increases or decreases. With those caveats in mind, the following characteristics are all positively associated with vegetation (Figure 14.1a):

1. *Density.* Vegetation density is similar to tissue density, as vegetation most often produces a level of brightness similar to myocardium; the greater the brightness (more similar to calcium), the less the likelihood that the echodensity is vegetation (though an old healed vegetation can be echo-bright).

2. *Size.* Vegetations can become quite large, especially in the setting of *Staphylococcus aureus* or fungal endocarditis. At the lower end, the limits of resolution for reliable identification of vegetation are 3 mm for TTE and 2 mm for TEE.

3. *Shape.* Vegetations tend to produce at least some irregularity and/or variability in shape (Figure 14.1b). Either the edges are fuzzy or friable, or the shape is amorphous, or the structure is multilobulated, or some combination of all of these characteristics.

4. *Location.* Vegetation almost always appears on the *upstream* or *regurgitant side of the valve* (i.e., the LVOT side for the aortic valve, within the LA for the mitral valve, and within the RA for the tricuspid valve).

5. *Mobility.* Vegetations tend to move in opposite symmetry to the valve opening and closing, and commonly will prolapse back and forth across the valve orifice.

6. *Associated complications.* These supportive findings include *flail leaflet, chordal rupture, abscess, fistula, pseudoaneurysm,* and in the case of prosthetic valves, *paravalvular leak and dehiscence.*

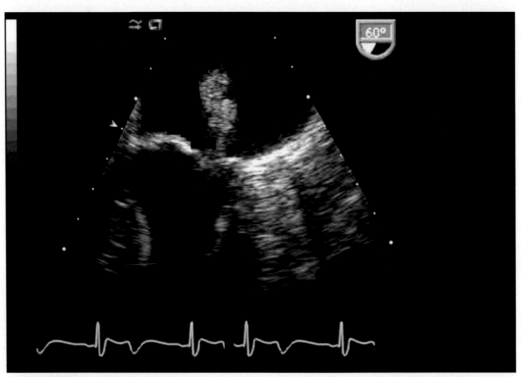

Figure 14.1a   TEE in the midesophageal view demonstrates a mitral valve vegetation on the "upstream" LA side of the valve.

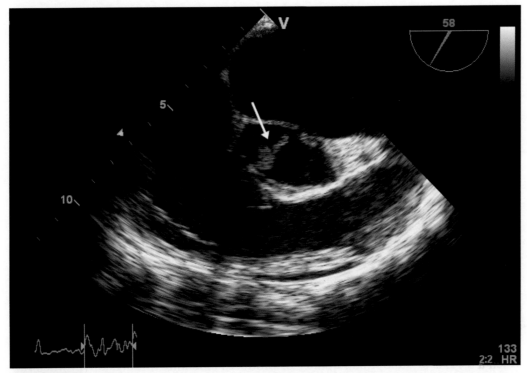

Figure 14.1b TEE demonstrates an irregularly shaped vegetation (arrow) covering the noncoronary cusp of the aortic valve.

The Diagnosis of Endocarditis

14.4 No single factor will make the diagnosis of endocarditis. The most commonly accepted method is to use a combination of clinical and echocardiographic criteria that produce high specificity. The *Duke criteria* accomplish these goals as well as any alternative, and thus are widely accepted (Table 14.1).

Table 14.1 Criteria for Endocarditis

Major	Minor
Multiple positive or persistently positive blood cultures	Predisposing heart disease or intravenous drug use
	Fever > 38°C
	Vascular phenomena
Positive echo findings:	Immunologic phenomena
Vegetation	Nondiagnostic echo findings
Infected device	Equivocal bacteriologic or serologic findings
Abscess	
Dehisced prosthesis	
New regurgitation	

Making the diagnosis according to the Duke criteria requires either two major criteria, one major plus three minor criteria, or five minor criteria. The criteria have several important implications for the echocardiographer. First, they establish that *the diagnosis of endocarditis can never be made solely on the basis of an echocardiogram.* By contrast, a combination of bacteriologic and immunologic criteria is sufficient even in the absence of echocardiographic findings (although it is not easy to do).

TTE Versus TEE for Diagnosing Endocarditis

14.5   Determining the proper test is an area that produces ongoing confusion, especially for the noncardiologist. Both tests have an important role to play, and both have strengths and weakness. While the sensitivity of TEE is superior to TTE (90% vs. 60% in aggregate studies), the specificity of both tests is similar at greater than 90%. TTE is a good test for making the straightforward diagnosis of native valve endocarditis in a patient who is otherwise clinically stable. If a high-quality TTE is negative, especially in the absence of valvular regurgitation, the incremental value of TEE is minimal (< 5%). Conversely, if diagnostic criteria are met and lead to a decision for medical therapy, TEE is unnecessary. The situations in which TEE is most valuable are (1) when a TTE is of suboptimal quality or produces indefinite findings or (2) when further clinical decision making depends critically upon echocardiographic findings. The outline in the following section implies that TEE is seldom a first-line diagnostic test, with the notable exception of prosthetic valve endocarditis. The one situation in which TEE utility is limited is when both an aortic and a mitral prosthesis are present, since the mitral prosthesis obscures visualization of the aortic prosthesis.

14.6   The following guidelines discuss when to use TTE and when to use TEE for the diagnosis and management of infective endocarditis. These guidelines are adapted from a 2008 report by the American College of Cardiology and the American Heart Association (adapted from *Circulation* Oct 2008;118:e523–e661, with permission). Most of the recommendations are based on Level of Evidence (no randomized or clinical trials, but judgment of experts).

Class I Indications (conditions for which there is evidence for and/or general agreement that the procedure or treatment is beneficial, useful and effective) for TTE in Endocarditis

1.   Detect valvular vegetations with or without positive blood cultures. (Level of Evidence: B)

2.   Characterization of the hemodynamic severity of valvular lesions in known infective endocarditis. (Level of Evidence: B)

3.   Assessment of complications of infective endocarditis (e.g., abscesses, perforation, and shunts). (Level of Evidence: B)

4.   Reassessment of high-risk patients (e.g., those with a virulent organism, clinical deterioration, persistent or recurrent fever, new murmur, or persistent bacteremia). (Level of Evidence: C)

Class IIa Indications (weight of evidence/opinion is in favor of usefulness/efficacy) for TTE in Endocarditis

Diagnosis of infective endocarditis of a prosthetic valve in the presence of persistent fever without bacteremia or a new murmur. (Level of Evidence: C)

Class IIb (usefulness/efficacy is less well established by evidence/opinion)

Reevaluation of prosthetic valve endocarditis during antibiotic therapy in the absence of clinical deterioration. (Level of Evidence: C)

Class III (conditions for which there is evidence and/or general agreement that the procedure/treatment is not useful/effective and in some cases may be harmful)

TTE is not indicated to reevaluate uncomplicated (including no regurgitation on baseline echocardiogram) native valve endocarditis during antibiotic treatment in the absence of clinical deterioration, new physical findings, or persistent fever. (Level of Evidence: C)

Class I Indications for TEE in Endocarditis

1. Assessment of the severity of valvular lesions in symptomatic patients with infective endocarditis, *if TTE is nondiagnostic.* (Level of Evidence: C)

2. Diagnosis of infective endocarditis in patients with valvular heart disease and positive blood cultures, *if TTE is nondiagnostic.* (Level of Evidence: C)

3. Diagnosis of complications of infective *endocarditis with potential impact on prognosis and management* (e.g., abscesses, perforation, and shunts). (Level of Evidence: C)

4. *First-line diagnostic study to diagnose prosthetic valve endocarditis and assess for complications* [italics added]. (Level of Evidence: C)

5. Preoperative evaluation in patients with known infective endocarditis, unless the need for surgery is evident on TTE and unless preoperative imaging will delay surgery in urgent cases. (Level of Evidence: C)

6. Intraoperative TEE for patients undergoing valve surgery for infective endocarditis. (Level of Evidence: C)

Class IIa

Diagnosis of possible infective endocarditis in patients with persistent staphylococcal bacteremia without a known source. (Level of Evidence: C)

Class IIb

Detection of infective endocarditis in patients with nosocomial staphylococcal bacteremia. (Level of Evidence: C)

14.7 *Echocardiographic predictors of mortality or adverse outcome in endocarditis*: Echocardiographic findings by either TTE or TEE that usually lead to valve replacement or an adverse outcome, regardless of clinical status include:

- *Vegetation size*. The embolic complication rate increases significantly at > 10 mm, or in the setting of rapidly expanding vegetation.

- *Valve failure*. Types of failure include flail leaflet, new severe regurgitation, or other deterioration of valve structure.

- *Abscess* (Figure 14.2) or *fistula formation*

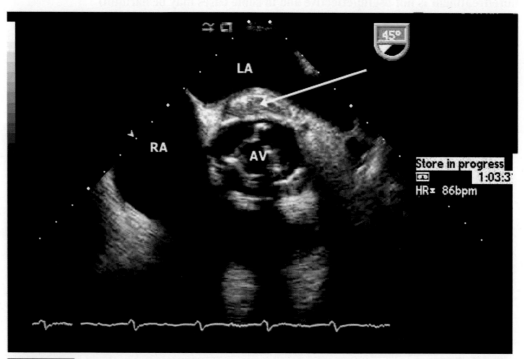

Figure 14.2   TEE midesophageal level of a bioprosthetic aortic valve (AV) demonstrates a large perivalvular abscess (arrow).

Prosthetic Valve Evaluation

14.8   Although the echogenicity of most prostheses presents a formidable set of challenges, echocardiography (Doppler in particular) still provides the best available tool for evaluation of prosthetic heart valves. Valve types include: ball and cage; tilting disc(s); porcine heterograft; and homograft, allograft conduit, and ring annuloplasty.

Ball and cage valves (e.g., Starr-Edwards [Figures 14.3a and 14.3b]) were widely used in the 1960s and 1970s. This type of valve has largely disappeared from the clinical scene but produces a characteristic echocardiographic appearance that identifies its presence with intense echogenicity. It is the most obstructive of prostheses.

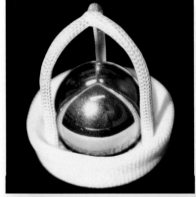

Figure 14.3a   (Left) Ball and cage (Starr-Edwards) valve. *Source*: Courtesy of the Office of History, NIH Stetten Museum.

Figure 14.3b   (Below) TTE two-chamber view shows the echodense profile of a Starr-Edwards mitral valve prosthesis (arrow).

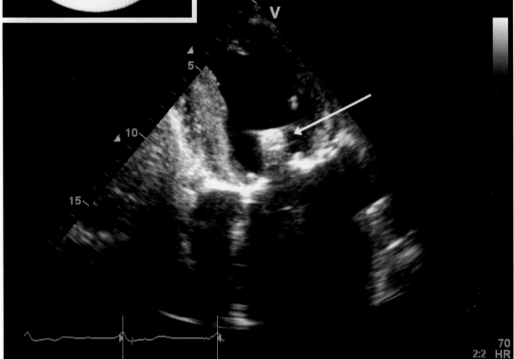

14.9   *Tilting disc valves* come in several forms, including single disc (e.g., Bjork-Shiley, Medtronic Hall [Figures 14.4a–14.4c]) or bileaflet discs (e.g., St. Jude [Figures 14.5a–14.5c], Carbomedics), with varying hinge points. The echo-reflectivity of both the discs and the surrounding housing varies with the materials used, but all of them tend to produce intense reverberation artifact. The angle of opening (90° for double-tilting disc valves) is a bit steeper than for single discs (80°). Both types produce a characteristic pattern of "physiologic" regurgitation with several jets that can readily be identified by TEE early in systole. Normal regurgitant volume for both valves varies from 5 to 10 ml. Cloth-covered sewing rings are used for both valves.

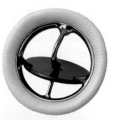

Figure 14.4a (Right) Medtronic Hall single-tilting disc heart valve. *Source*: Copyright Medtronic, Inc.

Figure 14.4b (Below) TEE midesophageal view demonstrates a Medtronic Hall single-disc mitral valve open in diastole. Note the large single leaflet (arrow).

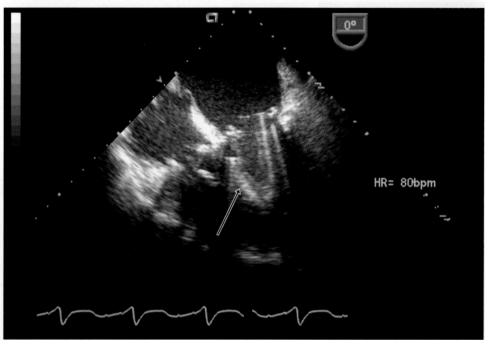

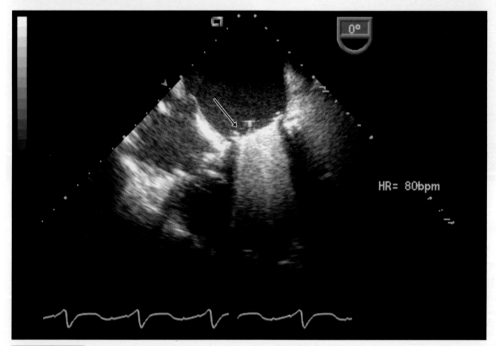

Figure 14.4c TEE midesophageal view demonstrates the same valve as in Figure 14.4a in systole. Fresh sutures (just placed in the operating room) are visible on the valve's atrial side (arrow). Intense reverberation artifact is produced by the single leaflet.

Figure 14.5a (Right) Regent™ Mechanical Heart Valve. A bileaflet heart valve. *Source*: Regent™ is a trademark of St. Jude Medical, Inc. Reprinted with permission of St. Jude Medical™, © 2010 All rights reserved.

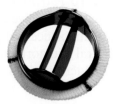

Figure 14.5b (Below) TEE midesophageal view demonstrates a St. Jude bileaflet mitral valve open in diastole. Note the reverberation artifact caused by both discs.

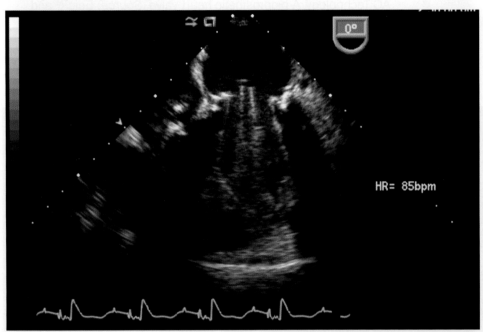

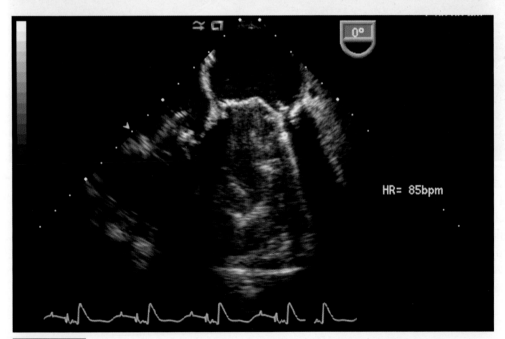

Figure 14.5c TEE midesophageal view systolic image demonstrates the St. Jude bileaflet mitral valve with closed leaflets.

14.10 *Porcine heterograft valves* (Figures 14.6a–14.6b) suspend a glutaraldehyde-fixed tissue valve over a three-pronged strut. The struts protrude well into the downstream orifice and produce a characteristic echocardiographic appearance in both the mitral and aortic positions as a pair of thick 2- to 3-mm parallel echodense lines. The echodensity of the struts limits visualization of the valve.

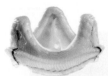

Figure 14.6a   (Left) Epic™ Supra Stented Tissue Valve with Linx™ AC Technology. A bioprosthetic heart valve. *Source*: Epic™ and Linx™ are trademarks of St. Jude Medical, Inc. Reprinted with permission of St. Jude Medical™, © 2010 All rights reserved.

Figure 14.6b   (Below) TTE in the apical four-chamber view of a mitral valve bioprosthesis. Note the supporting struts (arrow).

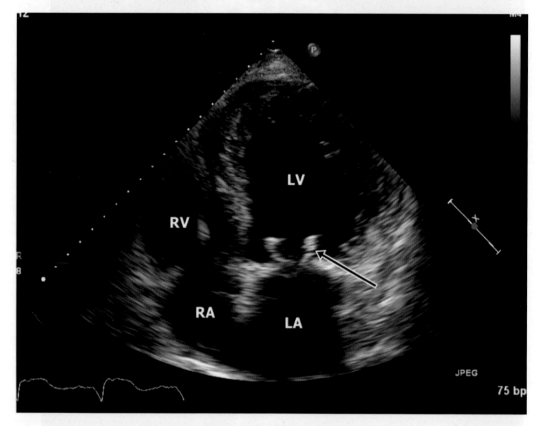

14.11 *Homografts, allograft conduits, and ring annuloplasty*: Aortic homografts come as a combined valve and conduit and are inserted as a unit. They are used in a variety of clinical settings, including younger adult patients who wish to avoid chronic anticoagulation and aortic dissection repair. They have the advantage of a normal hemodynamic profile, and they produce an echocardiographic appearance similar to a native valve and root. Pulmonic allografts are used for aortic valve replacement (Ross procedure) in congenital heart disease, with a homograft placed in the pulmonic position.

Their particular advantage was thought to be allowance for continued growth as the child ages and a decrease in the need for frequent repeat aortic valve replacement. More recently, their durability has been called into question.

Valve repair with or without the placement of an annuloplasty ring has emerged as a favored alternative to mitral valve replacement. Ring annuloplasty is also commonly used for tricuspid valve repair. The mitral ring can be well seen in the parasternal long axis view as a symmetrical echodensity on either side of the mitral annulus (Figure 14.7). The valve leaflets often appear be displaced apically.

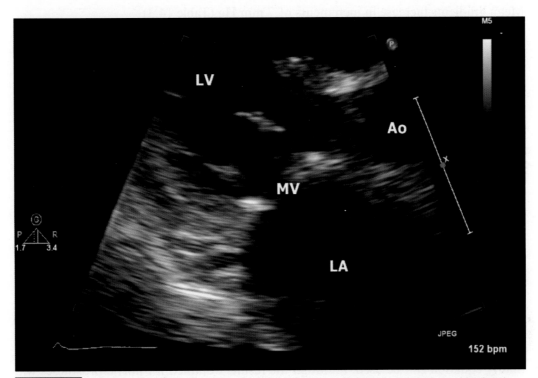

Figure 14.7   TTE in the parasternal long axis view demonstrates a mitral annuloplasty ring and valve repair in close-up in diastole, with typical displacement of the repaired mitral leaflets toward the apex.

Evaluation of Prosthetic Valve Function

14.12 Except for homografts, all other prosthetic valves are inherently stenotic, resulting in gradients above "normal." For normal prosthetic aortic valve velocities, think in terms of increasing in multiples of 5 mm Hg (Table 14.2). The dimensionless index for all types should be 0.3 or greater.

Table 14.2 Normal Peak Velocities for Prosthetic Aortic Valves

Valve Type	Peak Velocity
Homograft	2.0 m/sec
Tilting discs (e.g., Bjork-Shiley, St. Jude) and bioprostheses (e.g., Carpentier-Edwards)	2.5 m/sec
Starr-Edwards	3.0 m/sec

Mean gradients increase in increments of 7 mm Hg (Table 14.3).

Table 14.3 Normal Mean Gradients for Prosthetic Aortic Valves

Valve Type	Mean Gradient
Homograft	7 mm Hg
Tilting discs (e.g., Bjork-Shiley, St. Jude) and bioprostheses (e.g., Carpentier-Edwards)	14 mm Hg
Starr-Edwards (ball and cage)	23 mm Hg

For mitral prostheses, peak velocities for all types should be ≤ 2 m/sec, and mean gradients should be ≤ 5 mm Hg.

14.13 Because the echo-reflective properties of prosthetic heart valves often make direct visualization of valve function difficult, you must frequently rely on the available hemodynamics for assessment of valvular function. For mitral valve prostheses, the pressure half-time method will *overestimate* the mitral valve area. The original constant, 220, was derived from experience with rheumatic valves and does not match the characteristics of prosthetic valves. For both aortic and mitral prostheses, the continuity equation can be used, although the results obtained for aortic prostheses will overestimate aortic valve area slightly because of pressure recovery (see Section 7.4). For mitral prostheses, the equation functions in a manner similar to that employed for mitral stenosis:

$$\text{prosthetic mitral valve (MV) inflow} = \text{LVOT valve outflow}$$

$$\text{prosthetic (MVA)(VTI}_{MV}) = (\text{area}_{LVOT})(\text{VTI}_{LVOT})$$

$$\text{prosthetic MVA} = \frac{(0.785)(D_{LVOT})^2(\text{VTI}_{LVOT})}{\text{VTI}_{MV}}$$

This calculation depends upon measurements that can usually be made accurately without interference from the prosthesis.

A regurgitant mitral prosthesis will produce hemodynamics consistent with increased flow across the valve as a result of the regurgitant volume. Peak flow velocity will be increased beyond the normal prosthetic range to values of 2.5 m/sec or more, but pressure half-time will be normal or short (< 120 msec). Aortic flow, as measured by VTI_{LVOT}, will remain normal because it does not include mitral regurgitant volume.

14.14 *Patient prosthesis mismatch*: A smaller effective orifice area (EOA) after valve replacement compared to the native valve is not uncommon and usually is well tolerated. In a certain subset of patients, however, the decrease in EOA will be great enough to cause symptoms of fatigue or exercise intolerance. To estimate the value for a given patient, calculate the EOA with the continuity equation, using the flow and area of the unaffected valve. Use the outer diameter of the sewing ring for the diameter of the prosthetic valve and VTI. Then normalize the EOA of the valve to body surface area (BSA). The minimally acceptable value below which patient prosthesis mismatch may prove clinically significant is 0.85 cm²/m². EOA values < 0.6 cm²/m² are considered severe, are associated with excess mortality, and may lead to a recommendation for repeat valve replacement.

ADVANCED QUESTIONS

Q14.4   In a patient with a mechanical mitral prosthesis, determination of the degree of mitral regurgitation as determined by color Doppler flow by TTE is often limited by the acoustic shadow produced by the valve. Assuming the patient's LV function is otherwise normal, which of the following findings indicate the presence of severe prosthetic mitral regurgitation?

  a. Peak mitral valve inflow velocity of 3 m/sec, pressure half-time of 400 m/sec, VTI_{LVOT} of 25 cm

  b. Peak mitral valve inflow velocity of 3 m/sec, pressure half-time of 60 m/sec, VTI_{LVOT} of 30 cm

  c. Peak mitral valve inflow velocity of 1.5 m/sec, pressure half-time of 60 m/sec, VTI_{LVOT} of 30 cm

  d. Peak mitral valve inflow velocity of 1.5 m/sec, pressure half-time of 120 m/sec, VTI_{LVOT} of 20 cm

  e. Peak mitral valve inflow velocity of 1 m/sec, pressure half-time of 60 m/sec, VTI_{LVOT} of 70 cm

Q14.5   Which of the following patients has an absolute indication to undergo TEE for evaluation of endocarditis?

  a. A 25-year-old with a long history of intravenous drug use with staphylococcal bacteremia and a 4-mm vegetation identified on the anterior tricuspid leaflet who is otherwise clinically stable

  b. A 45-year-old with fever, urosepsis, and a holosystolic murmur

  c. A 65-year-old man with a septic joint following knee replacement, bacteremia, and a normal cardiac exam

  d. A 75-year-old man with a porcine aortic prosthesis and *Streptococcus viridans* bacteremia

  e. An 85-year-old man with known enterococcal endocarditis who is completing a six-week course of antibiotic therapy

Q14.6 What valve in the aortic position produces the highest mean pressure gradient?

a. Ball and cage

b. Single-tilting disc

c. Double-tilting disc

d. Porcine heterograft

e. Homograft

Q14.7 A 73-year-old woman who is six months post bioprosthetic aortic valve replacement presents with severe exertional dyspnea. Physical exam reveals clear lung fields and no edema. Echocardiography demonstrates normal biventricular systolic function, a transmitral E/A ratio < 1, E/E′ ratio of 7, and slight predominance of the systolic component of pulmonary venous flow. Estimated pulmonary artery systolic pressure is 40 mm Hg. TTE evaluation of the aortic valve prosthesis reveals no abnormalities. The patient's blood pressure is 125/70 mm Hg. Estimated body surface area is 1.5 m². LVOT diameter measured at the outer border of the sewing ring is 1.6 cm. LVOT VTI is 30 cm, and aortic valve VTI is 68 cm. You recommend:

a. Diuresis

b. Fluid bolus

c. Stress echocardiography

d. Pulmonary function testing

e. Repeat aortic valve replacement with a larger-diameter valve

Q14.8 The most accurate method for assessment of bioprosthetic mitral valve area is:

a. Pressure half-time

b. Direct planimetry by TEE

c. Subtraction of aortic outflow from mitral inflow

d. Continuity equation using aortic VTI_{LVOT} and D_{LVOT} diameter valve in the numerator and VTI_{MV} in the denominator.

e. Vena contracta width

Q14.9   Use of the continuity equation for evaluation of prosthetic valve function will:

a. Accurately estimate mitral valve area but overestimate aortic valve area

b. Underestimate aortic valve area and overestimate mitral valve area

c. Overestimate both aortic valve area and mitral valve area

d. Underestimate both aortic valve area and mitral valve area

e. Accurately estimate both aortic valve area and mitral valve area

ANSWERS

Q14.4 b: The high-peak mitral valve inflow velocity with a short pressure half-time suggests high-volume mitral valve inflow without mitral stenosis. A normal VTI_{LVOT} suggests that much of that flow is going backward through a regurgitant valve. Choice a suggests prosthetic mitral stenosis. Choices c and d suggest normally functioning valves. Choice e is high output from a nonvalvular cause. (Section **14.13**)

Q14.5 d: Bacteremia in the presence of a prosthetic valve is a Class I indication for TEE. (Section **14.6**)

Q14.6 a: These valves are increasingly rare in current practice, in no small part because of their unfavorable hemodynamic profile and inherent thrombogenicity. (Section **14.12**)

Q14.7 e: This is a case of patient prosthesis mismatch. First, calculate the prosthetic aortic valve area using the continuity equation, substituting the sewing ring diameter for the normal D_{LVOT}:

$$\text{Prosthetic aortic valve area} = 0.785(\text{sewing ring outer diameter})^2 \frac{(VTI_{LVOT})}{(VTI_{AV})}$$

$$= (0.785)(1.6 \text{ cm}^2)\frac{(30 \text{ cm})}{(68 \text{cm})}$$

$$= (2 \text{ cm}^2)(0.44)$$

$$= 0.9 \text{ cm}^2$$

Now divide the prosthetic aortic valve area by the BSA:

$$\frac{0.9 \text{ cm}^2 = 0.6}{1.5 \text{ cm}^2}$$

This is the cutoff for severe patient prosthesis mismatch. The rest of the data provided in this question is extraneous. (Section **14.14**)

Q14.8 d: See Section **14.13**.

Q14.9 a: The presence of pressure recovery, which is prominent with prosthetic aortic valves, will mean that prosthetic aortic valve area calculated by the continuity equation is slightly overestimated compared to results obtained by catheterization. Mitral valve area can be accurately estimated using the LVOT outflow and diameter. (Sections **14.13** and **7.4**)

15 ISCHEMIC HEART DISEASE

PRACTICE QUESTIONS

Q15.1 Which of the following standard views displays the portion of the interventicular septum supplied by the posterior descending artery?

a. Parasternal long axis

b. Parasternal short axis at the level of the papillary muscles

c. Apical four-chamber

d. Apical three-chamber

e. Apical five-chamber

Q15.2 What is the minimum stenosis required to cause a detectable wall motion abnormality during ischemia produced by stress echocardiography?

a. 40%

b. 50%

c. 60%

d. 80%

e. 90%

Q15.3   The still TEE image in Figure Q15.3 depicts:

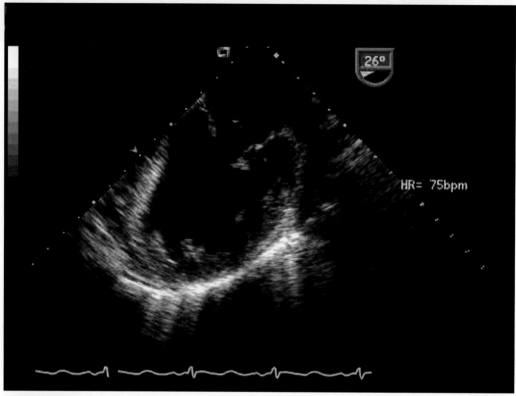

Figure Q15.3

    a. Ruptured chordae tendineae

    b. Ruptured papillary muscle

    c. Ruptured mitral leaflet

    d. Ruptured ventricular septum

    e. Ruptured LV free wall

ANSWERS: 15.1. c; 15.2. b; 15.3. b

15.1   Ischemic heart disease is by far the most common condition seen by cardiologists of adult patients. Essential knowledge begins with mastery of the relation between coronary distribution and wall segments, as outlined on an ASE wall motion map. The map is duplicative in that the parasternal views and apical views overlap (Figures 15.1a and 15.1b). The parasternal short axis view of the LV can be divided into three separate slices to demonstrate basal, mid-, and apical views, producing a 16-segment map. The apical four-chamber and two-chamber views are combined with the parasternal long axis view to produce a complementary 17-segment map that includes apical cap.

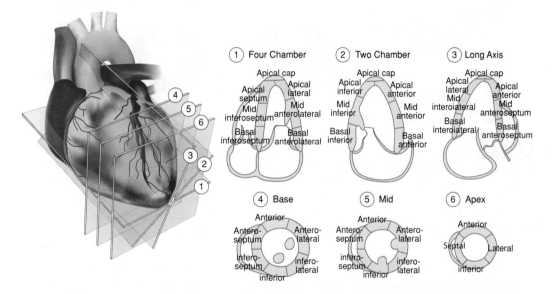

Figure 15.1a   Schematic of components of the ASE wall motion map. *Source*: Lang RM, Brierig M, et al. Recommendations for Chamber Quantification: A Report from the American Society of Echocardiography's Guidelines and Standards Committee and the Chamber Quantification Writing Group, Developed in Conjunction with the European Association of Echocardiography, a Branch of the European Society of Cardiology. *J Am Sc Echocardiogr*, 2005. 18:12;24.

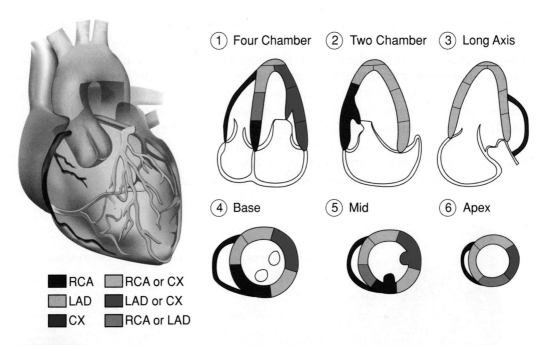

Figure 15.1b Relationship between individual wall segments and coronary artery distribution. *Source*: Lang RM, Brierig M, et al. Recommendations for Chamber Quantification: A Report from the American Society of Echocardiography's Guidelines and Standards Committee and the Chamber Quantification Writing Group, Developed in Conjunction with the European Association of Echocardiography, a Branch of the European Society of Cardiology. *J Am Sc Echocardiogr*, 2005. 18:12;24.

The left anterior descending artery supplies the anterior half of the septum, the anterior wall and apex, and, occasionally, the distal portion of the inferolateral wall and the distal RV free wall. The left circumflex artery supplies the lateral wall. The right coronary artery supplies the basal and midinferolateral wall, the basal and midinferior wall, and the proximal one-third of the septum via the posterior descending artery. In 10% of patients, the posterior descending artery is supplied by the left circumflex artery.

15.2 An *LV wall motion score* is constructed by grading each of the 17 segments on a 1–4 scale as follows:

- Normal = 1

- Hypokinetic = 2

- Akinetic = 3

- Dyskinetic = 4

Each of the 17 segments is graded, the scores are totaled, and the total is divided by the number of graded segments. A normal wall motion score would be 1 (17/17). In the setting of acute myocardial infarction, a wall motion score of greater than 1.7 is associated with an increase in cardiac events, such as hospitalization for heart failure, as well as increased mortality.

Complications of Coronary Artery Disease Readily Identified by Echocardiography

15.3   *Ventricular septal rupture* (Figures 15.2a and 15.2b) is a relatively rare event in the revascularization era. It typically occurs 3–7 days after myocardial infarction and commonly produces major clinical complications including heart failure and/or shock. The diagnosis can frequently be made by TTE and almost always by TEE. It should be suspected in any patient who after ST-elevation myocardial infarction develops a new systolic murmur or acute decompensation.

LEARNING DIRECTIVE

See Clip 15.32: Color flows left to right through the rupture, producing acute RV (and consequently LV) volume overload.

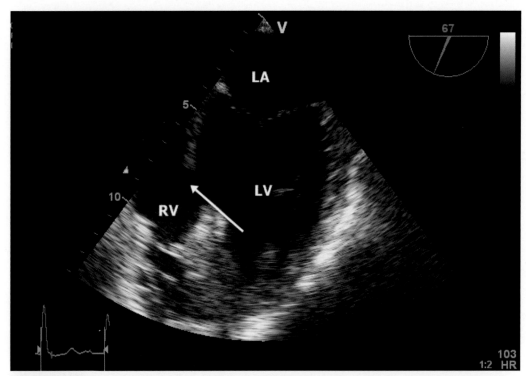

Figure 15.2a TEE demonstrates ventricular septal rupture (arrow).

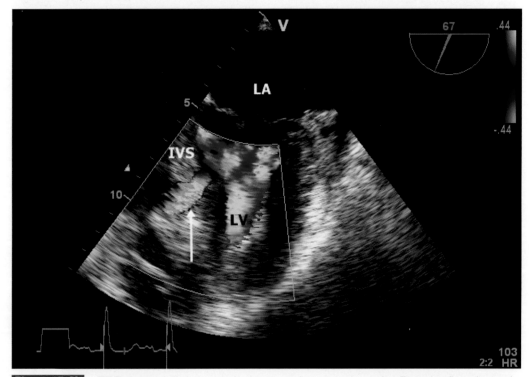

Figure 15.2b TEE demonstrates ventricular septal rupture by color Doppler flow (arrow). IVS, interventricular septum.

15.4 *Acute mitral regurgitation secondary to papillary muscle rupture* (Figure 15.3) has an epidemiology similar to ventricular septal rupture but is much more common in the setting of an inferior wall myocardial infarction because of the single blood supply to the posteromedial papillary muscle. Acute mitral regurgitation is almost always a major emergency that requires timely surgical repair. The degree of clinical instability depends upon the level of the rupture. Identification of a structural cause for mitral regurgitation is imperative because it determines that surgery will be required. Mitral regurgitation that is the result of ischemia may respond to percutaneous coronary revascularization.

LEARNING DIRECTIVE

See Clip 15.35: A broad jet of severe mitral regurgitation courses along the posterior atrial wall. The mitral regurgitation jet flows away from the affected mitral valve leaflet.

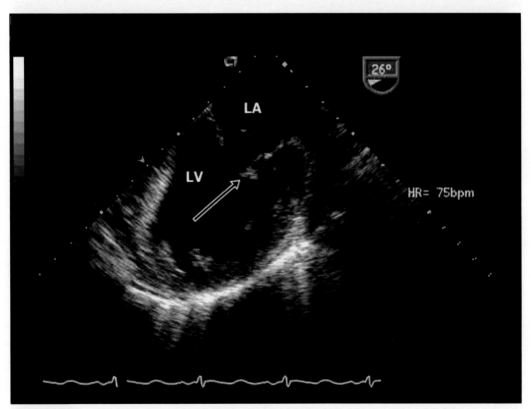

Figure 15.3   TEE in midesophageal view demonstrates acute papillary muscle rupture. The papillary muscle head (arrow) is separated from its attachment.

15.5 *Free wall rupture*: We have no clips of this catastrophe to display for an obvious reason—it is a fatal event. Because there has been no opportunity for ischemic preconditioning, free wall rupture is usually associated with a first myocardial infarction and single-vessel disease. Occasionally, the rupture will seal over and take the form of its cousin, *pseudoaneurysm*, in which the free wall is sealed off by a pericardial pouch (Figures 15.4a and 15.4b). Pseudoaneurysm is differentiated from true LV aneurysm by the presence of a narrow neck and to-and-fro flow through the channel. As a rule, urgent surgical repair is required and the associated mortality is fearsomely high, whether or not surgery is attempted.

> LEARNING DIRECTIVE
>
> **See Clip 15.40:** Ventricular pseudoaneurysm. Note the outer compartment of the aneurysm is created by the pericardium.

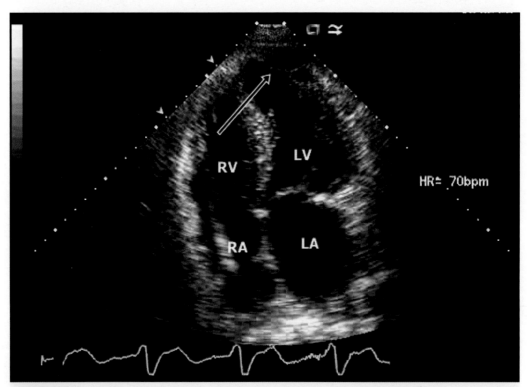

Figure 15.4a   TTE in the apical four-chamber view demonstrates ventricular pseudoaneurysm in the setting of an anterolateral wall myocardial infarction. Just beyond the thin membrane (arrow), the clear space of the pseudoaneurysm is seen.

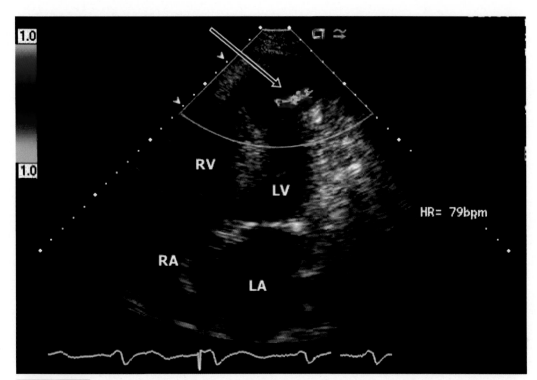

Figure 15.4b TTE in the apical four-chamber view demonstrates color flow through the narrow neck of the pseudoaneurysm (arrow).

Chronic complications of acute myocardial infarction include *ischemic mitral regurgitation.* The term ischemic mitral regurgitation is very much a misnomer. True ischemia leading to mitral regurgitation may be seen infrequently when normal papillary muscle function is impaired during exercise or any other condition that exacerbates reduced blood flow in the branch of the right coronary artery supplying the papillary muscle. In most cases, however, the mitral regurgitation is caused by a fixed structural defect or alteration in LV geometry as a consequence of previous myocardial infarction. Fixation or tethering, especially of the posterior leaflet, is a common factor. After myocardial infarction, even moderate mitral regurgitation in this setting (ERO 0.2–0.4 cm^2) is associated with a poor prognosis independent of ejection fraction.

LEARNING DIRECTIVE

See Clip 15.43: Ischemic mitral regurgitation.

15.6 *Echocardiogram predictors of poor prognosis following myocardial infarction* (in no particular order):

- LV ejection fraction $< 40\%$

- Decreased deceleration time (< 140 msec)

- Increased transmitral E/E$'$ (> 15)

- Wall motion score index > 1.7

- Mitral regurgitation with ERO > 0.20 cm^2

- LA volume index > 32 ml/m^2

15.7 *Stress echocardiography for ischemia*: Stress exercise echocardiography is an excellent technique for evaluation of ischemia and total coronary artery disease burden. The accumulated published experience demonstrates competitive sensitivity and predictive accuracy compared to nuclear imaging, with values greater than 85%. The threshold stenosis required to produce a detectable wall motion abnormality is widely reported at 50%. Nuclear imaging demonstrates slightly greater sensitivity, whereas stress echocardiography produces slightly higher specificity. Both sensitivity and specificity predictably increase with disease burden as defined by the number of vessels involved.

15.8 *Diastolic dysfunction is the most sensitive measure of ischemia.* The ischemic cascade begins with diastolic dysfunction. Suppose you have a dog fully instrumented in the (dog) catheterization lab. You have a pigtail catheter in place to measure LV end-diastolic pressure, an ECG to look for ST depression, a nuclear camera or similar device to look for change in perfusion, and an echocardiogram machine to look at wall motion. And, oh yes, we almost forgot, your dog talks! You place an angioplasty balloon in the dog's left anterior descending artery and watch what happens. The order of events is as follows:

1. The nuclear perfusion camera demonstrates reduced perfusion.

2. The pigtail catheter registers an abnormality as LV end-diastolic pressure rises.

3. The echocardiogram machine registers an anterior wall motion abnormality.

4. The ECG shows ST depression.

5. Lastly, the dog says, "Arf, arf! Take this balloon catheter out of my artery. My chest is killing me!"

The point of this attempt to humorously describe what is classically referred to as the "ischemic cascade" is to reinforce the notion that wall motion is a highly sensitive measure of ischemia, even more so than the potassium channel leak responsible for ST depression, and certainly more so than the sensation of angina. That fact makes stress echocardiography a powerful indicator of ischemia even in the absence of other findings.

The technique is not without limitations. Its accuracy is completely dependent upon the quality of the pictures obtained and thus upon the skill of the sonographer. After 60 seconds postexercise, the ability to detect ischemia decreases precipitously, and even that is a generous window depending upon the maximum heart rate achieved. Bicycle exercise offers an alternative that is not as operator dependent because scanning can be performed continuously during exercise.

15.9 *Dobutamine stress echocardiography* is a superior test for the assessment of cardiovascular risk for noncardiac surgery and for determination of prognosis in anticipation of revascularization. Patients with myocardial viability exhibit a *biphasic response*, showing transient improvement in contractility with low doses of dobutamine and worsening with high doses (Table 15.1). The presence of a biphasic response predicts a favorable outcome after revascularization, in which a repeat resting echocardiogram will resemble the low-dose dobutamine images. Conversely, lack of a biphasic response predicts poor prognosis and poor surgical outcome.

Table 15.1 Wall Motion Response to Dobutamine

Dose	Rest	Low	High	Recovery
Normal	NL	↑	↑↑	NL
Ischemia	NL	NL/↓	↓↓	↓
Infarct/Scar	↓	↓	↓↓	↓
Viable/Hibernating	↓	↑	↓↓	↓

ADVANCED QUESTIONS

Q15.4   Which of the following statements regarding myocardial viability as determined by dobutamine stress echocardiography is true?

    a.   The presence of viability provides no information regarding prognosis.

    b.   Viable myocardium is the result of severely restricted coronary blood flow.

    c.   Atropine is required to demonstrate myocardial viability.

    d.   A biphasic response to dobutamine infusion indicates myocardial scar.

    e.   Improvement after revascularization is common in all myocardial segments.

Q15.5   Which variable predicts *decreased* survival after myocardial infarction?

    a.   Transmitral E/E' ratio of 8

    b.   LV end-systolic volume of 40 ml

    c.   Increased LA volume index (> 32 cm^2/m^2)

    d.   An LV wall motion score of 1.5

    e.   An LV ejection fraction of 45%

Q15.6   What is the temporal order of ischemic-induced abnormalities observed during stress echocardiography?

    a.   Increased LV end-diastolic pressure, abnormal LV wall motion, ST depression, angina

    b.   Abnormal LV wall motion, ST depression, angina, increased LV end-diastolic pressure

    c.   Angina, abnormal LV wall motion, increased LV end-diastolic pressure, ST depression

    d.   ST depression, increased LV end-diastolic pressure, angina, abnormal LV wall motion

    e.   Increased LV end-diastolic pressure, ST depression, abnormal LV wall motion, angina

Q15.7 The presence of new mitral regurgitation is a marker of adverse prognosis after:

a. Pulmonary embolism

b. Acute myocardial infarction

c. Endocarditis

d. Coronary artery bypass surgery

e. Percutaneous patent foramen ovale closure

Q15.8 A patient presents with an extensive new inferior wall myocardial infarction. TTE demonstrates dyskinesis of the basal inferior and inferolateral walls; akinesis of the basal septal, midinferior, and inferolateral walls; and hypokinesis of the distal inferior wall. The remaining walls contract normally. What is the patient's wall motion score?

a. 1

b. 1.5

c. 1.7

d. 1.8

e. 2.0

Q15.9 The wall motion score in the previous question:

a. Predicts LV ejection fraction

b. Predicts increased risk for repeat hospitalization and repeat cardiac events in the year following the infarction

c. Predicts LA size

d. Predicts total exercise tolerance following myocardial infarction

e. Predicts viability with dobutamine echocardiography

ANSWERS

Q15.4   b: Viable myocardium is tissue in which blood flow is present but severely restricted. Viability provides powerful information regarding prognosis following revascularization. Viability is usually demonstrated at low doses of dobutamine. A biphasic response is characteristic. Only viable segments will demonstrate improvement. (Section **15.9**)

Q15.5   c: Increased LA volume index is a predictor of increased events and decreased survival following acute myocardial infarction, as well as a predictor of recurrent atrial fibrillation following cardioversion. The factors mentioned also predict adverse outcomes following myocardial infarction, but not at the cutoffs listed. (Section **15.6**)

Q15.6   a: This is the proper ordering of the ischemic cascade. Section **15.8**.

Q15.7   b: Even new moderate mitral regurgitation (ERO > 0.2 cm^2) is associated with poorer outcomes. (Section **15.6**)

Q15.8   d

- Two segments are dyskinetic: $2 \times 4 = 8$

- Three segments are akinetic: $3 \times 3 = 9$

- One segment is hypokinetic: $= 1 \times 2 = 2$

- The remaining segments are normal: $11 \times 1 = 11$

- Wall motion score (total points divided by 17): $30/17 = 1.8$

(Section **15.2**)

Q15.9   b: A wall motion score > 1.7 is a predictor of recurrent hospitalization and recurrent events following acute myocardial infarction. (Section **15.2**)

16

CARDIAC MASSES

For Questions 16.1–16.6, match the cardiac tumor with its most common location.

    a. Fibroma

    b. Angiosarcoma

    c. Papillary fibroelastoma

    d. Rhabdomyoma

    e. Myxoma

    f. Hypernephroma

Q16.1 RA

Q16.2 LV wall

Q16.3 RV or LV cavity

Q16.4 Aortic valve

Q16.5 Inferior vena cava

Q16.6 LA

ANSWERS: 16.1. b; 16.2. a; 16.3. d; 16.4. c; 16.5. f; 16.6. e

---

Primary Neoplasms

16.1 *Myxoma* is the most common primary cardiac tumor. Although it is most frequently found within the LA (Figure 16.1), it may also be found within the RA (Figure 16.2) or ventricular locations. In rare cases, such as familial myxoma syndromes, there may be multiple sites. The tumor has a polyploid irregular appearance. Symptoms include dyspnea, orthopnea, paroxysmal nocturnal dyspnea, pulmonary edema, cough, hemoptysis, edema, and fatigue. Patients may present with stroke due to migration of the tumor or overlying thrombus. Myxoma most often has a stalklike septal attachment but may originate from any endocardial surface. The tumor is notorious for embolizing or may cause syncope as the result of direct obstruction to mitral or tricuspid valve inflow. Myxoma can be part of a rare familial syndrome known as the *Carney complex*, which presents with lentigines and hormone-secreting tumors.

LEARNING DIRECTIVE

See Clip 16.1: A left atrial myxoma in the four-chamber view.

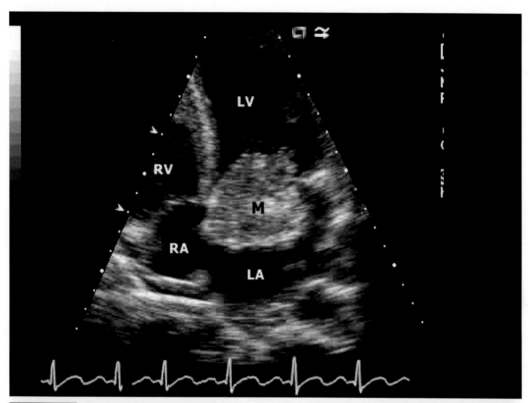

Figure 16.1 TTE in the apical four-chamber view demonstrates a large LA myxoma (M) obstructing mitral inflow.

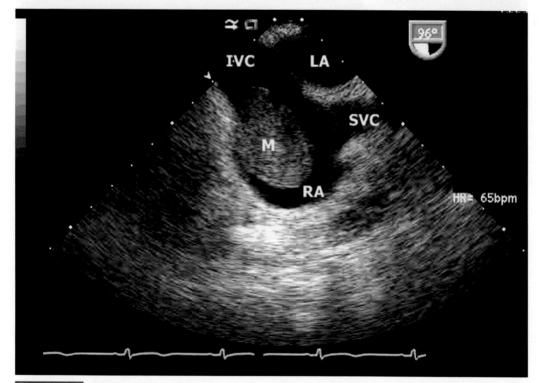

Figure 16.2 TEE in the midesophageal view demonstrating the myxoma's (M) attachment site within the RA free wall. SVC, superior vena cava; IVC, inferior vena cava.

16.2   *Fibromas* are usually intramuscular and are often found in the LV free wall. If the tumor expands sufficiently, it can produce obstruction. Fibromas are associated with lethal cardiac arrhythmias.

16.3   *Papillary fibroelastomas* (Figures 16.3a and 16.3b) usually present as round, mobile masses on a stalk attached to one of the aortic leaflets or another valve, but they may emerge from any endocardial surface. Single or multiple fibroelastomas may be present. While histologically benign, a papillary fibroelastoma may embolize as it enlarges, and removal is recommended.

LEARNING DIRECTIVE

See Clip 16.6: A papillary fibroelastoma attached to the right coronary cusp.

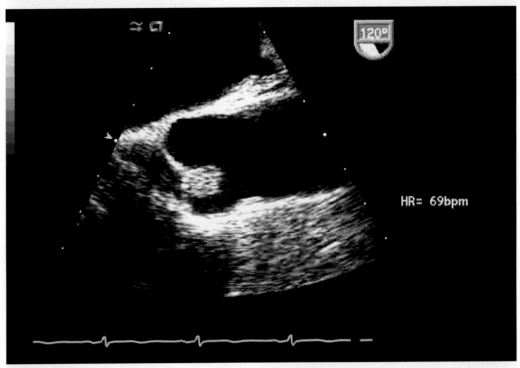

Figure 16.3a   TEE in a midesophageal view at 120° demonstrates papillary fibroelastoma (arrow) on the aortic valve.

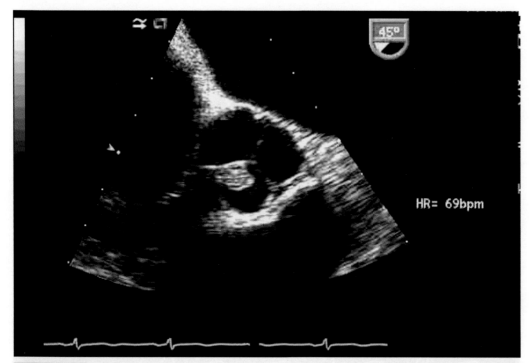

Figure 16.3b   TEE in a midesophageal view in the same patient demonstrates a papillary fibroelastoma (arrow). This cross-sectional view identifies the location as the right coronary leaflet (RC). LC, left coronary leaflet; NC, noncoronary leaflet.

16.4   *Angiosarcomas* (Figure 16.4) are aggressive invasive tumors with a predilection for the *RA* (80%). More frequent in men, angiosarcomas are the most common primary malignant neoplasm in adults and are usually fatal.

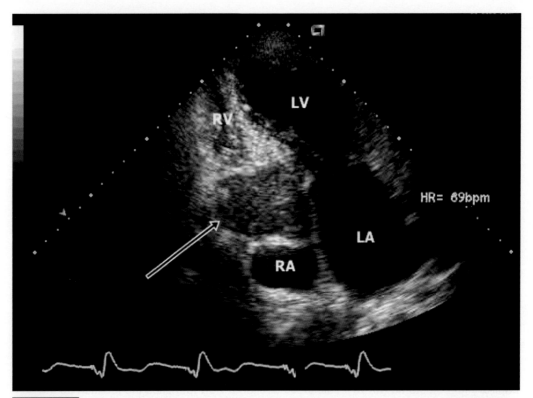

Figure 16.4 TEE in an apical four-chamber view demonstrates a large echogenic mass (arrow) causing near total obliteration of the RA. On biopsy, the mass proved to be an angiosarcoma.

16.5 *Rhabdomyomas* are benign tumors that are seen in children and often regress (Figure 16.5). The tumors may present singly or in multiple forms and are usually located within the LV or RV cavities. In the multiple forms, they are associated with *tuberous sclerosis*.

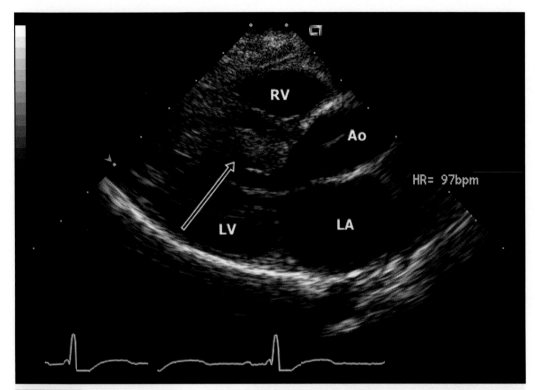

Figure 16.5   TTE in the parasternal long axis view demonstrates a large rhabdomyoma (arrow).

Metastatic Neoplasms

16.6   Metastatic tumors within the heart occur 20–40 times more frequently than primary tumors. The four most common cancers that produce cardiac involvement, especially within the pericardium, are (in no particular order) *lung, breast, lymphoma,* and *melanoma.* Spread may occur hematogenously or by direct lymphatic extension depending upon tumor type and location. Cardiac metastases are often invasive. Melanoma, in particular, has a predilection for the heart, with 60% of metastatic disease demonstrating cardiac involvement, either pericardial or myocardial, or both. Though cardiac involvement is common in melanoma, it rarely results in tamponade or other compromise.

16.7   *Renal cell carcinoma* will extend directly into the inferior vena cava and may be observed in that location in the subcostal view (Figure 16.6).

See Clip 16.9: A large mass seen in the inferior vena cava. The differential diagnosis includes thrombus and renal cell carcinoma.

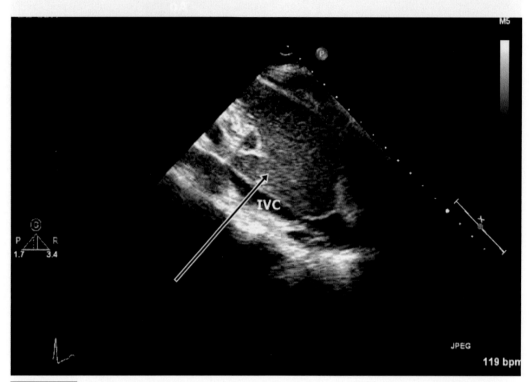

Figure 16.6   TTE subcostal view demonstrates a large mass (arrow) in a patient with renal cell carcinoma that nearly obliterates the inferior vena cava (IVC).

Other Masses

16.8   *Thrombus* is a common finding that occurs in a variety of settings that can be assessed echocardiographically:

1. As a complication of myocardial infarction or cardiomyopathy, in which the thrombus will involve the LV apex or forms a mural layer over the infarcted wall (Figures 16.7a and 16.7b). A contrast agent can be used to confirm the presence and location of the mass (Figure 16.7c).

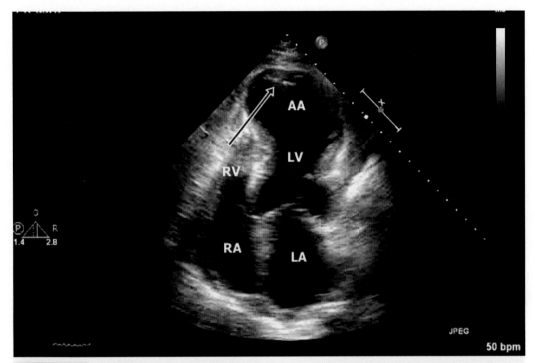

Figure 16.7a TTE from the apical four-chamber view demonstrates an apical mural thrombus (arrow) in the setting of an extensive anterior wall myocardial infarction with an apical aneurysm (AA).

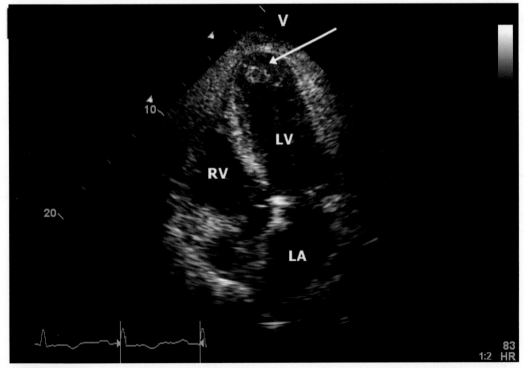

Figure 16.7b TTE from the apical four-chamber view demonstrates an apical thrombus (arrow).

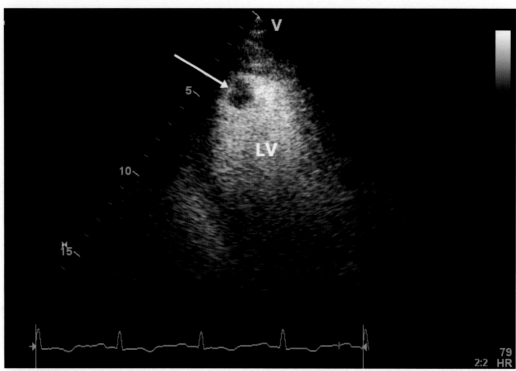

Figure 16.7c   TTE from the apical four-chamber view after administration of echo contrast in the same patient as in Figure 16.7b highlights the location and extent of the thrombus (arrow).

2. As a complication of atrial fibrillation, in which the thrombus forms within the *LA appendage* (Figures 16.8a and 16.8b). Spontaneous echocardiographical contrast and depressed LA appendage flow velocities (< 20 cm/sec) are a nearly universal feature in this setting, and RA thrombi, although rare, may also be seen. Detection of LA thrombus is best accomplished by TEE, which provides definitive guidance for safe cardioversion without prolonged anticoagulation beforehand.

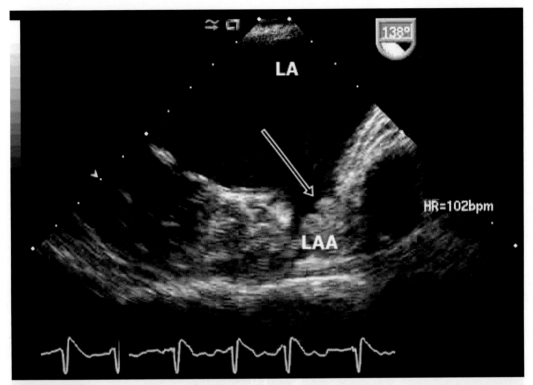

Figure 16.8a TEE from the midesophageal view demonstrates LA appendage thrombus at 138°.

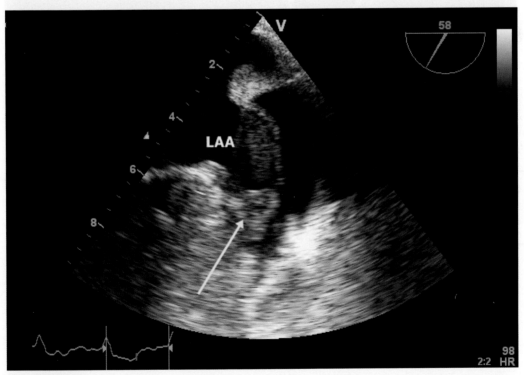

Figure 16.8b TEE from the midesophageal view demonstrates an apical LA appendage thrombus at 58°.

3. As a cause of pulmonary or paradoxical embolism. The diagnosis is mostly made by inference in the setting of a patent foramen ovale or atrial septal defect, but *thrombus in transit* may occasionally be seen (Figure 16.9), either through the right heart or, rather spectacularly, through the interatrial septum.

LEARNING DIRECTIVE

See Clip 16.12: Thrombus in transit in a patient with a recent pulmonary embolism.

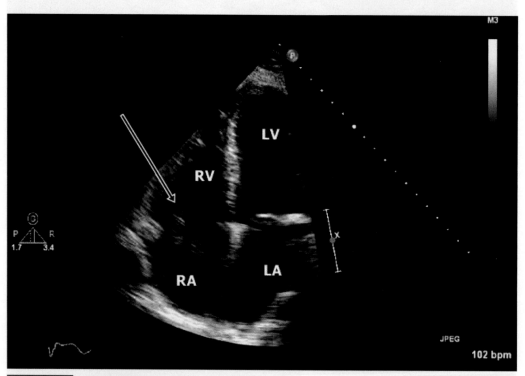

Figure 16.9 TEE in the four-chamber view demonstrates thrombus in transit through the tricuspid annulus (arrow).

Although thrombus produces an echodensity similar to myocardium, it can regularly be distinguished by its *location* (intra- or extracardiac), its shape (irregular, pedunculated, or popcorn-like if mobile; laminar if sessile, as with mural thrombus), its *noncongruent motion,* and its *lack of thickening* in contrast to normal myocardium. Thrombus size and mobility impact the likelihood that TEE evaluation will be required.

Normal Variants

16.9 The *eustachian valve* (Figure 16.10) is a remnant of the valve of the fetal inferior vena cava that directs oxygenated blood toward the foramen ovale. The *Chiari network* (Figure 16.11) is a filamentous membrane of similar origin. The size, echodensity, and mobility of either structure may vary greatly, but the attachment site for both structures will be at or near the junction of the inferior vena cava and the RA. In the appropriate clinical setting, the differential diagnosis for both structures includes thrombus and tumor as described previously. Neither structure is pathologic.

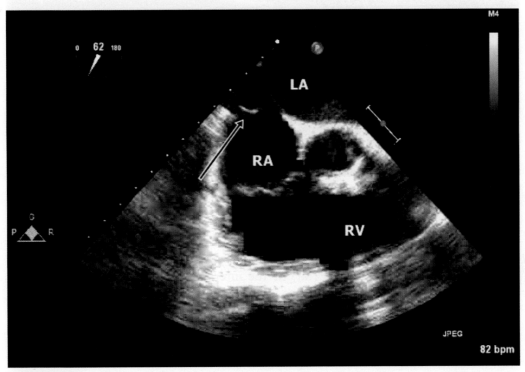

Figure 16.10 TEE in midesophageal view of the RA demonstrates of a eustachian valve (arrow).

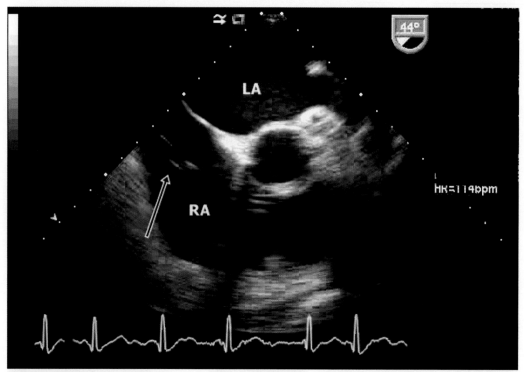

Figure 16.11 TEE in the midesophageal view of the RA demonstrates a Chiari network (arrow).

16.10 *Lipomatous septal hypertrophy of the interatrial septum* (Figure 16.12) appears as moderate-intensity thickening (fat) of the interatrial septum with sparing of the fossa ovalis in a "dumbbell" appearance. Although there is a possible association with patent foramen ovale, lipomatous hypertrophy is a benign phenomenon.

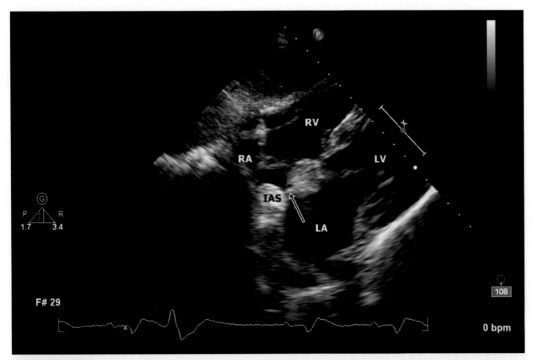

Figure 16.12 TTE in the subcostal view demonstrating lipomatous hypertrophy of the interatrial septum (IAS). The septum has a dumbbell shape, and there is sparing of the fossa ovalis (arrow).

16.11 *Lambl's excrescences* (Figure 16.13) are small (2–4 mm) mobile filamentous strands seen on the downstream side of the aortic valve and less commonly the mitral valve leaflets. They are believed to be formed as fibrin deposits overlaid by an initial layer of intimal cells that ultimately condense and separate from the valve surface.

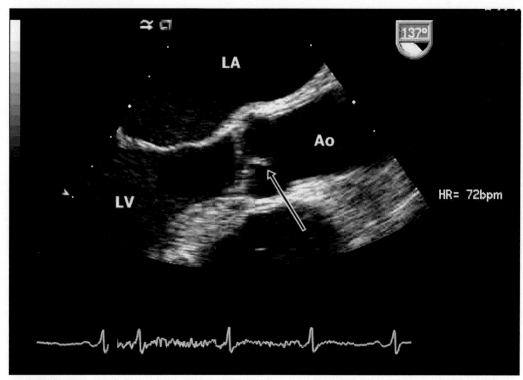

Figure 16.13   TEE at the midesophageal level demonstrating Lambl's excrescences (arrow).

16.12 *External masses* may produce hemodynamic compromise, depending upon their location, and can often be observed by echocardiography. Intrapericardial thrombus following cardiac surgery may commonly produce external compression and tamponade physiology. Hiatal hernia with retained gastric contents may compress the LA and produce hypotension (Figure 16.14). The true nature of the "mass" can sometimes be characterized by having the patient drink a carbonated beverage.

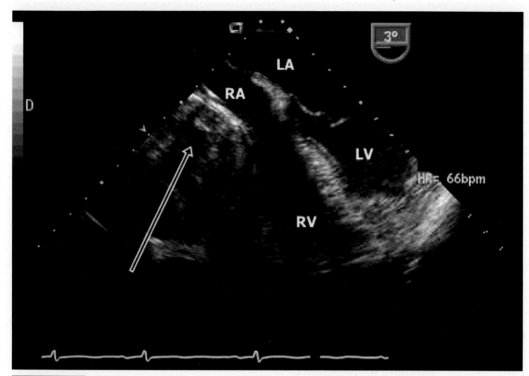

Figure 16.14 TEE in the midesophageal view demonstrates the presence of an external mass causing RA compression.

ADVANCED QUESTIONS

Q16.7   Which tumor is associated with lethal cardiac arrhythmias?

    a. Fibroma

    b. Angiosarcoma

    c. Papillary fibroelastoma

    d. Rhabdomyoma

    e. Myxoma

For Questions 16.8–16.10, match the skin finding with the tumor.

    a. Fibroma

    b. Angiosarcoma

    c. Papillary fibroelastoma

    d. Rhabdomyoma

    e. Myxoma

Q16.8   Lentigenes

Q16.9   Facial angiofibromas in a butterfly distribution

Q16.10   Café-au-lait spots

ANSWERS

Q16.7   a: Fibroma is associated with an increased risk of malignant arrhythmias and sudden cardiac death. (Section **16.2**)

Q16.8   e: Lentigenes are part of the Carney complex associated with a small portion of patients with myxoma. (Section **16.1**)

Q16.9   d: Facial angiofibromas are one of the manifestations of tuberous sclerosis, which is also associated with rhabdomyoma. (Section **16.5**)

Q16.10   d: Café-au-lait spots are another of the manifestations of tuberous sclerosis, which is associated with rhabdomyoma. (Section **16.5**)

17

ECHOCARDIOGRAPHY IN SYSTEMIC DISEASE

PRACTICE QUESTIONS

Q17.1 Aortic regurgitation is a well-described clinical and echocardiographic feature of which of the following diseases?

   a. Ankylosing spondylitis

   b. Ehlers-Danlos syndrome, type 4

   c. Freidrich ataxia

   d. Hypereosinophilia

   e. Fabry disease

Q17.2 Fenfluramine, a drug used previously for weight loss, produces which of the following echocardiographic abnormalities?

   a. Aortic stenosis

   b. Restrictive cardiomyopathy

   c. Mitral regurgitation

   d. LV aneurysm

   e. Pericardial effusion

ANSWERS: 17.1. a; 17.2. c

17.1 A number of diseases with cardiac involvement produce characteristic echocardiographic findings. Though not extensive, the following list includes the most common disorders.

Hypereosinophilic syndrome produces apical infiltration of eosinophils and thrombus as well as mitral leaflet thickening and immobility (Figure 17.1).

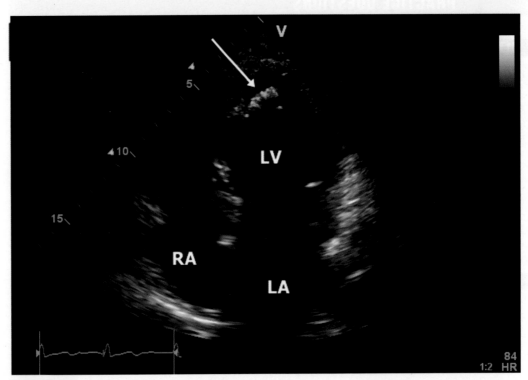

Figure 17.1 TTE apical four-chamber view demonstrates apical thrombus (arrow) in a patient with hypereosinophilic syndrome.

Sarcoidosis produces posterobasalar aneurysm and regional wall motion abnormalities mimicking coronary artery disease. Thinning of the basal anterior septum has also been described. Sarcoidosis can also produce a nonspecific cardiomyopathy.

Ankylosing spondylitis produces aortic regurgitation from aortic root dilation. The mechanism of the aortic regurgitation is directly related to the aortic abnormalities.

Systemic lupus erythematosus produces pericardial effusion, aortitis, aortic insufficiency, and Libman-Sacks endocarditis. Libman-Sacks vegetations preferentially involve the tips of the mitral leaflets and may be relatively symmetrical (Figure 17.2). They rarely reach more than 10 mm in diameter and are sessile. In contrast to infectious vegetations, independent motion is not seen.

LEARNING DIRECTIVE

See Clip 17.4: Libman-Sacks endocarditis in a patient with systemic lupus erythematosus. Note the characteristic nonmobile thickening at the tips of the anterior and posterior mitral leaflets.

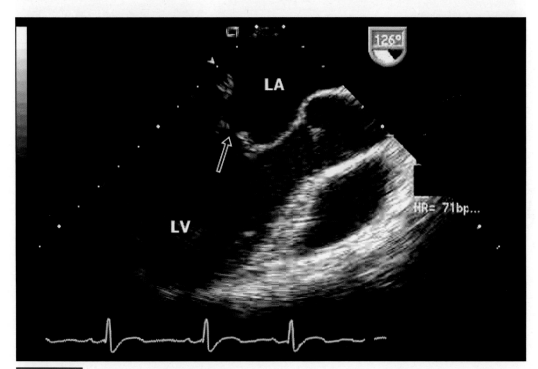

Figure 17.2 TEE in a midesophageal view demonstrates Libman-Sacks endocarditis (arrow).

Carcinoid produces pulmonic stenosis and tricuspid regurgitation (Figure 17.3). The tricuspid valve leaflets are characteristically fixed open in an immobile position. Most cardiac involvement is right sided because of filtration of serotonin by the lungs, but a small percentage of patients (< 10%) demonstrates left-sided findings as well.

LEARNING DIRECTIVE

See Clip 17.2: The immobility of the valve produces wide-open tricuspid regurgitation, one of the hallmarks of the disease.

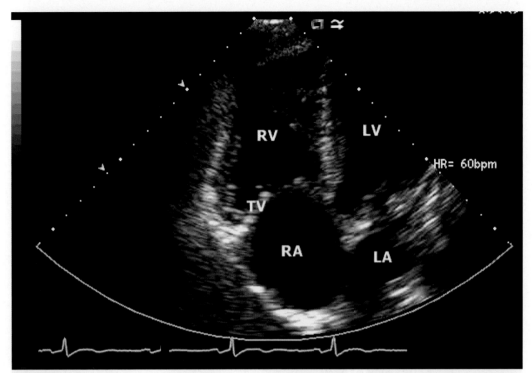

Figure 17.3 TTE in the four-chamber view demonstrates tricuspid valve (TV) involvement in carcinoid heart disease. Note the dilated RV as well.

Marfan syndrome produces aortic aneurysm, aortic dissection, and mitral valve prolapse. A dilated aorta is a critical criterion in making the diagnosis.

Friedreich ataxia produces LV hypertrophy.

Fabry disease (Figure 17.4) produces LV hypertrophy in the absence of hypertension or aortic stenosis with a characteristic linear echo-brightness along the endocardial border. Fabry disease has been found with a frequency of 3–4% in patients with unexplained LV hypertrophy. The diagnosis can be confirmed by a blood test for α-galactosidase.

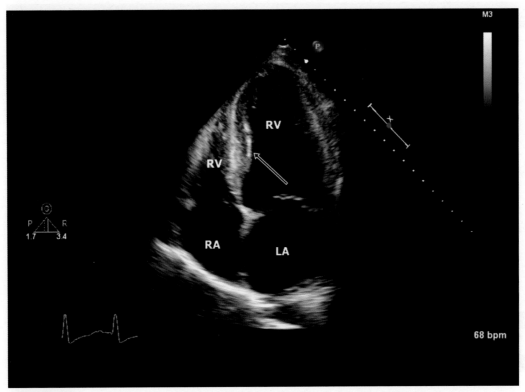

Figure 17.4   TTE in the four-chamber view in a patient with Fabry disease. The endocardial border assumes a characteristic linear brightness (arrow).

Rheumatoid arthritis produces pericardial effusion.

Scleroderma produces pulmonary artery hypertension, diastolic dysfunction, and aortic sclerosis.

Hemochromatosis can present as a dilated cardiomyopathy but otherwise offers no specific findings to aid in the diagnosis. Disease severity appears to be related to the degree of iron deposit present, which can often be assessed.

17.2   Drugs causing cardiac abnormalities detectable by echocardiography include procainamide, hydralazine, and minoxidil, which all produce pericardial effusion (lupus like syndrome).

Daunorubicin, cyclophosphamide, and other chemotherapeutic agents are associated with dilated cardiomyopathy. Fenfluramine, a serotonin analog, was used widely in the 1990s in combination with phentermine as an appetite suppressant for weight loss. In patients receiving the drug for prolonged periods (> 6 months), its serotonergic properties frequently produced varying degrees of mitral and/or aortic regurgitation. When mild, the regurgitation often reversed with cessation of the drug, but a small number of patients developed severe disease requiring valve replacement. The drug also caused accelerated, fatal pulmonary artery hypertension in a small number of patients.

ADVANCED QUESTIONS

For Questions 17.3–17.8, match the systemic disease with the echocardiographic finding.

a. Systemic lupus erythematosus

b. Marfan syndrome

c. Fenfluramine-phentermine use

d. Fabry disease

e. Hypereosinophilic syndrome

f. Sarcoidosis

Q17.3   Aortic dissection

Q17.4   Posterobasilar LV aneurysm

Q17.5   Apical LV thrombus

Q17.6   Reversible mitral regurgitation

Q17.7   LV hypertrophy

Q17.8   Noninfectious endocarditis

ANSWERS

Q17.3   b: Section 17.1.

Q17.4   f: Section 17.1.

Q17.5   e: Section 17.1.

Q17.6   c: Section 17.2.

Q17.7   d: Section 17.1.

Q17.8   a: Section 17.1.

18

AORTIC ANEURYSM, DISSECTION, HEMATOMA, AND ATHEROMA

PRACTICE QUESTIONS

Q18.1 Which of the following TEE findings has been identified as a likely cardiac source of embolism?

a. Isolated patent foramen ovale

b. Isolated atrial septal aneurysm

c. Aortic atheroma < 4 mm

d. Ulcerated aortic plaque

e. Spontaneous echocardiographic contrast in the LA appendage

Q18.2 What is the relative sensitivity and specificity for the diagnosis of aortic dissection by TEE compared to CT scan?

a. Sensitivity of TEE is higher, and specificity is lower.

b. Sensitivity of TEE is higher, and specificity is higher.

c. Sensitivity of TEE is lower, and specificity is higher.

d. Sensitivity of TEE is lower, and specificity is lower.

e. Both sensitivity and specificity of TEE are similar to CT scan.

Q18.3 In aortic dissection, which portion of the aorta is least visible by TEE?

a. Aortic root

b. Ascending aorta

c. Transverse arch

d. Descending aorta

e. Dissection is well seen throughout the aorta by TEE.

Aortic Dissection

18.1 Type A dissection is one of the most critical diagnoses that can be made by echocardiography. This is a surgical disease with a historic unoperated mortality of 1%/hour. While TTE has limited sensitivity for the diagnosis, it can often provide initial clues as to the presence of dissection, such as new aortic regurgitation or pericardial effusion. The proximal aorta, however, is a common site for linear reduplication artifacts that can mimic dissection, so care must be taken to avoid a false-positive diagnosis. True dissections will usually produce a clear border that undulates in synchronization with aortic motion, restricts color flow, and can be seen in several imaging planes.

LEARNING DIRECTIVE

See Clip 18.1: A parasternal long axis view suspicious for complex proximal dissection.

18.2 TEE remains a definitive test with unassailable advantages over other modalities. The test can be performed in almost any critical care setting without the need for additional monitoring or patient transfer. In the hands of a skilled operator, the diagnosis can be made almost as soon as the probe is passed into the esophagus, and TEE's sensitivity, specificity, and predictive accuracy are similar compared to competing modalities. Both proximal (type A, originating above the ligamentum arteriosum) and distal dissections (type B, originating below the ligamentum arteriosum) are well seen.

LEARNING DIRECTIVE

See Clip 18.5: Once again, color Doppler flow shows restriction of flow to the true lumen.

18.3 Dissection is well visualized in multiple planes (Figure 18.1).

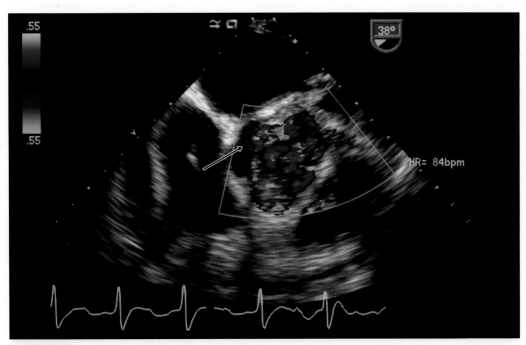

Figure 18.1 TEE midesophageal view at 38° demonstrates a proximal aortic dissection (arrow) into the noncoronary cusp (arrow) seen in a short axis orientation. The dissection flap excludes normal systolic flow as demonstrated by color Doppler.

The origin can often be determined by visualizing the aorta along its long axis in a vertical view (Figure 18.2a). Doppler color-flow interrogation will usually separate out the true and false lumen (Figure 18.2b).

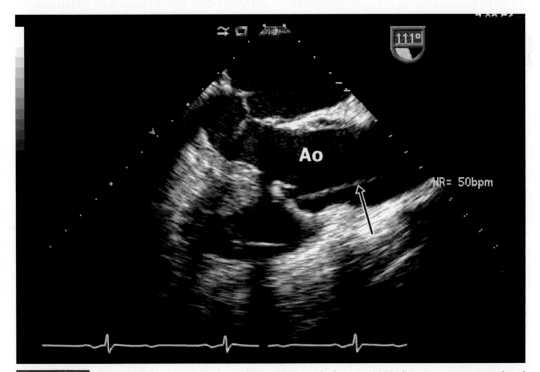

Figure 18.2a TEE of the aorta in the midesophageal view at 110° demonstrates proximal (type A) dissection (arrow) seen in long axis. The origin of the dissection can be seen within the aortic root.

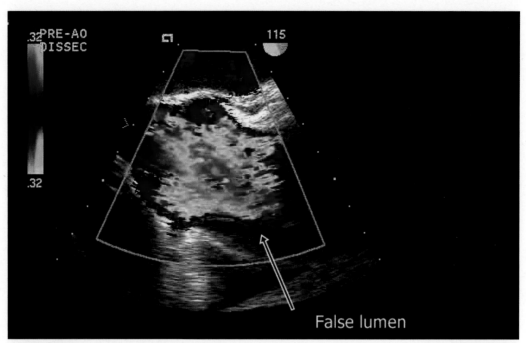

False lumen

Figure 18.2b   TEE of the aorta in the midesophageal view at 115° demonstrates color Doppler flow confined to the true lumen.

TEE's major disadvantage is its limited ability to visualize the proximal transverse arch because of the interposition of the trachea, so that the origin of type A or proximal dissection may be difficult to detect if it lies above the ligamentum arteriosum but beyond the ascending arch. Complications depend upon the direction of extension of the dissection and include stroke (extension into the left common carotid artery), acute myocardial infarction (extension into a coronary artery), and renal failure (extension into a renal artery). Extension into the aortic root may lead to leaflet prolapse and subsequent aortic insufficiency. Rupture into the pericardial space may produce cardiac tamponade.

18.4   *Aortic hematoma* is caused by rupture of the vasa vasorum with bleeding between the outermost aortic layer and the media. Subsequent thrombus formation extends into the aortic lumen, producing the hematoma. The hematoma, which produces the tissue density typical of thrombus (in contrast to the echo-free space produced by dissection), is separated from the true lumen by the intima. The hematoma usually produces a crescentlike appearance, and the circular shape of the aorta in cross section is usually preserved (Figure 18.3).

LEARNING DIRECTIVE
See Clip 18.8: Limited color Doppler flow through the lumen.

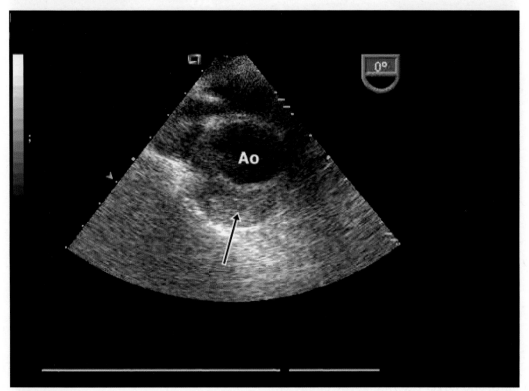

Figure 18.3   TEE of the descending thoracic aorta demonstrates aortic hematoma (arrow).

Similar to dissection, the thrombus may extend for a variable distance as the aortic planes are further separated (Figure 18.4).

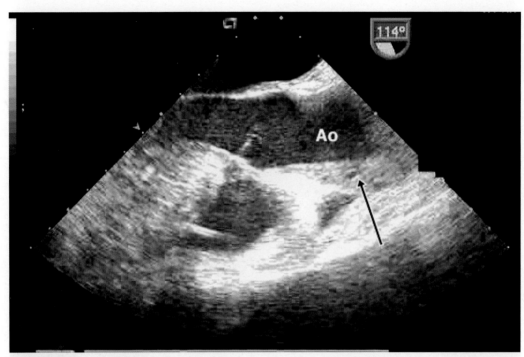

Figure 18.4 TEE in the midesophageal view at 114° demonstrates an aortic hematoma (arrow) extending from the aortic root along the proximal aorta.

TEE, CT, and MRI all provide superior diagnosing ability compared to aortography and TTE. Aortography can produce a false-negative result because of the absence of a false lumen. Aortic hematoma has a relentless tendency to progress to dissection with a similarly fearsome mortality. It is treated by surgical repair whenever possible. Risk of progression increases with proximal location, increased hematoma thickness (> 11 mm), and larger external aortic diameter.

18.5 *Aortic transection* occurs most commonly as a complication of high-speed deceleration injury as occurs in motor vehicle accidents. The ligamentum arteriosum serves as a fulcrum around which the aorta will tear in cross-section. If the rupture is confined, survival, however transient, will provide a narrow window of opportunity for aortic repair. The disruption of the aortic wall will produce a layer within the lumen that is thicker and less mobile than a dissection flap (Figure 18.5).

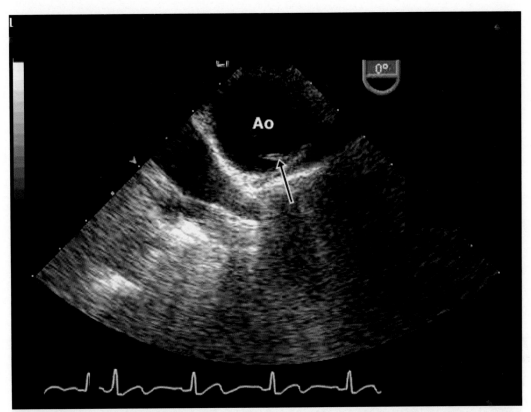

Figure 18.5 TEE of the descending aorta in cross-section demonstrates aortic transection (arrow).

LEARNING DIRECTIVE

See Clip 18.28: Color Doppler interrogation shows exclusion of flow outside the transection.

In complete transection, color Doppler flow will produce a characteristic double ring of bidirectional flow inside and outside the transection (Figure 18.6).

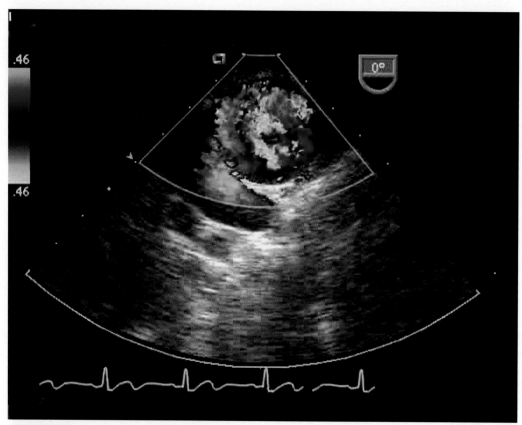

Figure 18.6   TEE of the descending aortic arch demonstrates color flow interrogation of aortic transection producing the characteristic "bulls eye" pattern.

18.6   *Penetrating atherosclerotic ulcer* represents an advanced manifestation of atherosclerotic vascular disease. The lesion erodes into the medial layer and produces a focal crater within the lumen (Figure 18.7). Penetrating ulcers are usually confined to the distal aorta and do not commonly extend.

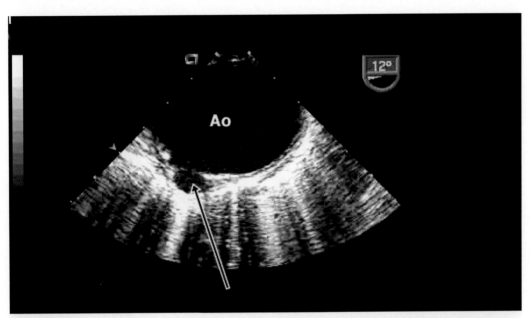

Figure 18.7   TEE of the descending thoracic aorta demonstrates a penetrating aortic ulcer (arrow) seen in cross-section.

18.7   *Aortic atheroma* is a frequent finding by TEE and presents a common cardiac source of embolism. Atheroma may be laminar or may penetrate into the lumen and be mobile (Figures 18.8a and 18.8b). Stroke risk increases significantly when the cross-sectional thickness of the atheroma exceeds 4 mm.

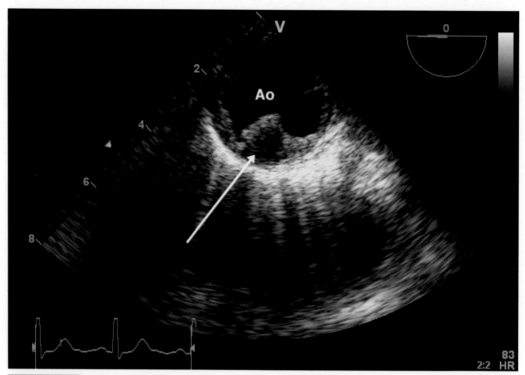

Figure 18.8a TEE of the descending thoracic aorta in short axis demonstrates complex atheroma (≥ 4 mm thick) (arrow).

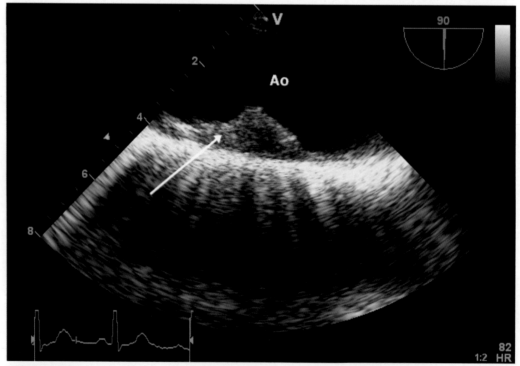

Figure 18.8b TEE of the same region of the descending thoracic aorta (Ao) in long axis demonstrates the extent of the atheroma (arrow).

Aortic Aneurysm

18.8 The dilation produced by true aortic aneurysms extends through all three aortic layers. The most common cause of aortic aneurysm, *cystic medial necrosis*, is largely a consequence of systemic hypertension and atherosclerotic vascular disease. *Aortitis* may produce focal, diffuse, or patchy dilation depending upon whether the etiology is inflammatory disease such as Takayasu or giant cell arteritis, or infection. *Syphilitic aortitis* produces extensive dilation emanating from the aortic root and is a rare finding in the antibiotic era. In patients with Marfan syndrome, aortic dilation may be focal or diffuse. Localization of dilatation to the sinuses is associated with a more favorable prognosis, whereas rapid progression of expansion and family history of severe cardiovascular complications predict a more ominous outcome.

True aneurysms may be *saccular* (as is the case with syphilitic aortitis) or *diffuse* as in sytemic hypertension.

Most proximal ascending aortic aneurysms are well seen by TTE. Aneurysm size can be followed quantitatively by serial 2D TTE measurements. For children and young adults, vessel diameter should be normalized for age and body surface area according to published nomograms available in the ASE quantification statement.

False aneurysms are produced by penetration into the intimal and medial layers of the aorta but not the adventitia, with flow back and forth in the fashion of pseudoaneurysms elsewhere. Trauma is the most prominent cause, and lesions produced in this circumstance have a high probability of progressing to dissection or complete rupture.

18.9 *Sinus of Valsalva aneurysm* appears as focal dilation of one or more of the sinuses. If the aneurysm is large enough, it may impinge upon or deform adjacent structures, especially the RV or RA (Figures 18.9a and 18.9b).

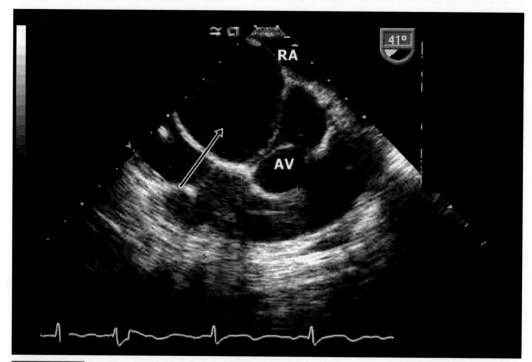

Figure 18.9a   TEE of the aorta in the midesophageal view at 41° demonstrates an aneurysm of the sinus of Valsalva of the right coronary cusp (arrow) displacing the RA.

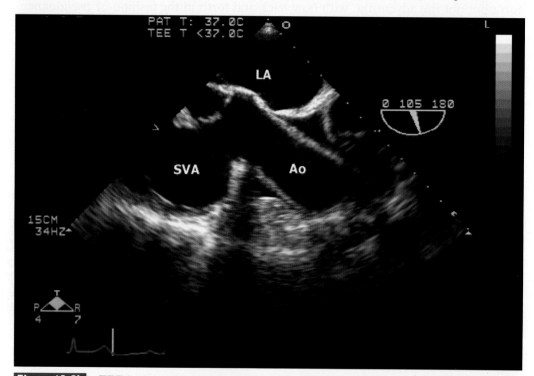

Figure 18.9b   TEE in the midesophageal view at 105° demonstrates a large right sinus of Valsalva aneurysm (SVA) in a longitudinal orientation.

Aortic regurgitation is a common complication. The aneurysm may rupture into the RV producing hemodynamics (and an echocardiographic appearance) similar to that seen with a ventricular septal defect, except that flow is continuous.

ADVANCED QUESTIONS

For Questions 18.4–18.7, match the description to the disease most closely associated with it.

a. Prognosis depends upon location and extent

b. A complication of syphilitic aortitis

c. Does not progress to dissection or rupture

d. Caused by rupture of the vasa vasorum

e. Will often displace the right atrium

f. Commonly caused by chest trauma

Q18.4   Saccular aneurysm

Q18.5   False aneurysm

Q18.6   Sinus of Valsalva aneurysm

Q18.7   Aneurysm secondary to Marfan syndrome

For Questions 18.8–18.12, match the description of risk to the correct condition.

a. The risk of a catastrophic event is 100%.

b. The risk of a catastrophic event is unpredictable.

c. The risk of a catastrophic event is location dependent.

d. The risk of a catastrophic event increases at ≥ 4 mm.

e. The risk of a catastrophic event increases at > 11 mm.

Q18.8   Aortic atheroma

Q18.9   Aortic hematoma

Q18.10   Penetrating aortic ulcer

Q18.11   Aortic transection

Q18.12   Aortic dissection

ANSWERS

Q18.4   b: For answers to Questions **18.4**–**18.7**, see Sections **18.8** and **18.9**.

Q18.5   f

Q18.6   e

Q18.7   a

Q18.8   d: For answers to Questions **18.8**–**18.12**, see Sections **18.3**–**18.7**.

Q18.9   e

Q18.10   b

Q18.11   a

Q18.12   c

19 RHYTHM EFFECTS

PRACTICE QUESTIONS

Q19.1 Which of the following echocardiographic findings is the strongest predictor of maintenance of sinus rhythm following cardioversion?

    a. Degree of mitral regurgitation

    b. RA volume

    c. Transmitral E/A ratio

    d. Pulmonary atrial flow velocity (PV_a) width

    e. LA appendage ejection velocity

Q19.2 Prolonged first-degree atrioventricular block produces what effect upon the transmitral E/A ratio?

    a. Peak E velocity increases, and peak A velocity decreases.

    b. Peak E velocity decreases, and peak A velocity increases.

    c. Peak E velocity increases, and peak A velocity increases.

    d. Peak E velocity decreases, and peak A velocity decreases.

Q19.3   The spectral Doppler tracing in Figure Q19.3 demonstrates:

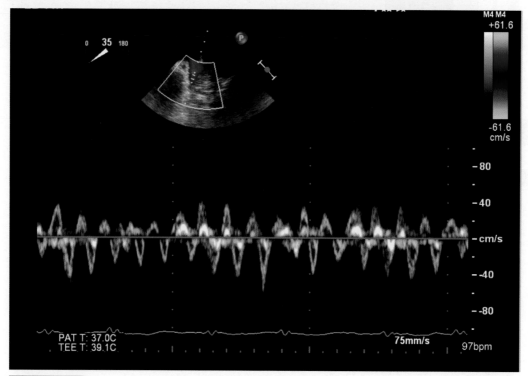

Figure Q19.3

a. Atrial fibrillation

b. Atrial flutter

c. Atrioventricular nodal reentry tachycardia

d. Ventricular tachycardia

e. Sinus tachycardia

19.1 Interrogation of the LA appendage by spectral Doppler during TEE produces a characteristic series of patterns depending upon the underlying rhythm. In sinus rhythm, the Doppler pattern reveals three components, with the largest jet moving toward the transducer in late systole during appendage contraction (Figure 19.1).

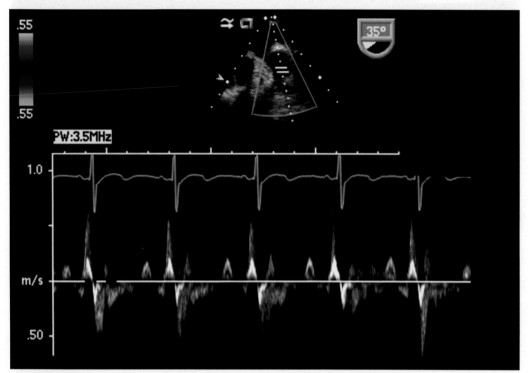

Figure 19.1 Spectral Doppler pattern of LA appendage flow in sinus rhythm.

In atrial fibrillation, coarse fibrillatory waves can be readily seen (Figure 19.2).

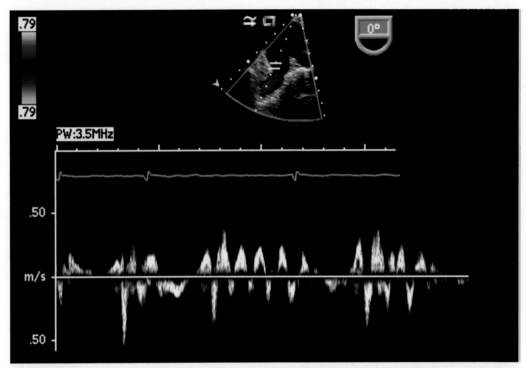

Figure 19.2   TEE midesophageal view of spectral Doppler interrogation of the LA appendage in a patient with atrial fibrillation demonstrating fibrillatory waves.

The peak velocity of the LA appendage fibrillatory waves is a powerful predictor of the ability to maintain sinus rhythm following cardioversion, with values < 50 cm/sec, as seen in Figure 19.2, predicting a poor response. Flutter waves will produce a more regular pattern, with the number of waves per RR interval matching the flutter rate (Figure 19.3).

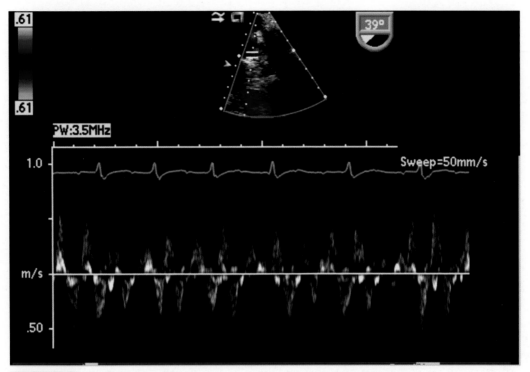

Figure 19.3 Spectral Doppler of atrial flutter waves in the LA appendage.

19.2 Intrinsic cardiac rhythm and alterations in atriovenrticular (AV) conduction produce a variety of echocardiographic and Doppler effects. Normal separation of the transmitral E and A waves depends upon sinus rhythm, and tachycardia may cause the E and A waves to fuse together. The PR interval also influences the relative height of the E and A wave. As the PR interval lengthens, the time available for atrial contraction increases, and the height of the A wave rises relative to the E wave. This phenomenon provides a key guide to manipulation of the atrioventricular delay during atrioventricular optimization of biventricular pacing. The atrioventricular interval is manipulated to produce the most optimal contribution of atrial filling or largest A wave relative to E wave. At short atrioventricular intervals, the E wave predominates because there is inadequate time to produce optimal atrial contraction. In Figure 19.4, note the pattern in this patient with an atrioventricular delay of 100 msec.

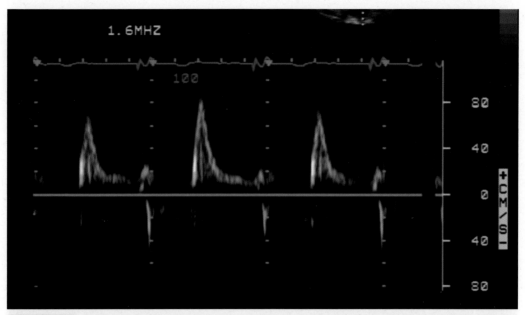

Figure 19.4   An atrioventricular interval at 100 msec increases the transmitral E/A ratio.

As the AV delay is lengthened, the relative height of the transmitral A wave is increased relative to the E wave, and total diastolic filling increases (Figure 19.5).

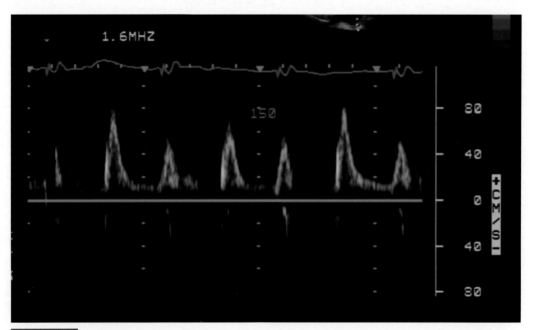

Figure 19.5   Increasing the atrioventricular interval to 150 msec increases atrial filling and reduces the transmitral E/A ratio.

During atrioventricular optimization, series of atrioventricular intervals are employed sequentially until the optimal effect is produced. Other parameters simultaneously evaluated in this setting include degree of mitral regurgitation stroke volume and cardiac output as measured by LV outflow tract VTI.

ADVANCED QUESTIONS

Q19.4   Patients with biventricular pacemakers often undergo atrioventricular optimization, in which the atrioventricular interval is adjusted to produce maximal cardiac output. Which set of echocardiographic variables is used most commonly for this purpose?

a.   Transmitral E/A ratio, stroke volume, degree of mitral regurgitation

b.   Transmitral E/A ratio, E/E′ ratio, stroke volume

c.   Transmitral E/A ratio, PV_a, degree of mitral regurgitation

d.   Transmitral E/E′ ratio, stroke volume, degree of mitral regurgitation

e.   Transmitral E/A ratio, PV_a, stroke volume

Q19.5   In patients with biventricular pacemakers, manipulation of the atrioventricular delay is commonly employed to optimize cardiac function. Which of the following echocardiographic parameters is assessed?

a.   Pulmonary vein spectral Doppler pattern

b.   Mitral inflow Doppler pattern

c.   End-diastolic dimension

d.   LV ejection fraction

e.   Septal-lateral wall delay measured by strain imaging

ANSWERS

Q19.4   a: Altering the atrioventricular interval properly will increase the transmitral A wave, thus improving stroke volume and reducing mitral regurgitation. (Section **19.2**)

Q19.5   b: This is an easier variant of Question 19.2. (Section **19.2**)

Front

NEW Patient

Patient Last/First Name, MRN, DOB
Echo Lab (E,S,W)
Height, weight, BP, Tape 08 XX-X:XX

Parasternal Long Axis
   2D, zoom, color Doppler, LVOT diam
   Anatomic M-mode: AoV/LA, MV, LV
RV Inflow: 2D, color, CW
RV Outflow: 2D, color, PW, CW
Parasternal Short Axis
   2D, color AoV, PValve, TValve
     Pulsed/CW PValve, TV
   Basal, Mid, Apical LV-2D
Apical 4 Chamber
   2D, color, pulsed/CW MV/TV
     Pulsed PVein
   VTI (>140 fps); spectral lat/sept walls
Apical 5 Chamber
   2D, color, pulsed LVOT; CW AoV
Apical 2 Chamber: 2D, color; VTI
Apical 3 Chamber: 2D, color, CW AoV; VTI
Subcostal 4Ch: 2D,color IAS, IVS, IVC, Ao
Suprasternal: 2D color, pulsed/CW Ao
Right Parasternal: 2D dil Ao, CW for AS

Back

Normal Reference Values
LA: PLA <4.1 cm; 4Ch <5.3 cm
      LA vol <28 ml/m^2
RA: 4Ch <5.1 cm
LV: Anteriorseptum <1.2 cm
      Inferolateral <1.2 cm
      EDD <5.7 cm
Effusion: Diastolic Small <1.0 cm; large >2.0 cm
RV: Supine EDD <2.2 cm
Aorta: Root <3.7 cm; Ascending <3.5 cm
      Arch <3.1 cm; Descending <2.6 cm
AoValve: nl velocity <2.0 m/s
LVOT velocity: nl <1.5 m/s
AoVArea = π(LVOT$_{diam}^2$)(LVOT$_{vel}$)/4*AoV$_{vel}$
  AS: Mild >1.2; Mod 1–1.2; Sev <1.0 cm^2
  AR P$_{1/2}$: Mild >500; vena contracta $\leq$0.3 cm
    Mod 350–500; Mod–sev 200–350
    Severe <200 ms, vena contracta $\geq$0.6 cm
Mitral Valve: **MVA** = 220/P$_{1/2}$ time
  MS: P$_{1/2}$ time: = 0.29*decel time
    Mild >1.5; Mod 1.0–1.5; Sev <1.0 cm^2
  MR: Mild 20%; ERO <0.2; Sev $\geq$40%; ERO $\geq$0.40
E wave decel: 140–250 ms
E/E´: < 8(nl); >15 (LEVDP >18 mmHg)
PV velocity: nl <1.5m/s
TR velocity: nl <2.5m/s
Mod Bernoulli: ΔPressure = 4V^2

7/28/09 v3

BETH ISRAEL DEACONESS MEDICAL CENTER

Boston, Massachusetts 02215

Name:

DOB: **Medical Record Number:**

Addressograph:

Date **Indication for TEE:**

/ / Brief History:

Pertinent PMHx:

TEE Safety: Esoph/GI, NPO

Medications:

Allergies:

Focused Physical Examination

BP ___ /___   HR ___ /min   Rhythm: SR AF

Airway: Mallampati Class:

Lungs

Heart:

Risks and benefits of the procedure explained. All questions answered.
Permission granted to proceed with TEE. Signed consent in chart. Reviewed
with attending staff.

_____, MD _____, MD

TEE Fellow Beeper#   Attending Beeper #

INFORMED CONSENT FOR TRANSESOPHAGEAL ECHOCARDIOGRAPHY

BETH ISRAEL DEACONESS MEDICAL CENTER

Boston, Massachusetts 02215

CONSENT FOR TRANSESOPHAGEAL ECHOCARDIOGRAM

Addressograph:_____ (name of healthcare provider) has explained that I have a condition called _____ (name of condition) and has recommended a medial or surgical treatment called transesophageal echocardiography.

Benefits and Alternatives to Treatment: My doctor has spoken with me about the benefits I may expect from this treatment, such as _____ diagnosis of_____ but has made no guarantees or promises. My doctor has also spoken about what could happen if I do not get this treatment and explained other options for my care, including ____decline of the procedure.

Risks: My doctor has explained that there are some risks to this treatment. The risks include, but are not limited to, allergic reactions, drug reactions, bleeding, blood clots, nerve injury, brain damage, infection, loss of bodily function or life, or the need for more procedures or treatments. My doctor has also explained that there may be other risks or complications. Particular risks include, but are not limited to : ___ perforation of the esophagus or stomach, low or high blood pressure, bleeding, damage to the vocal cords, hoarseness, sore throat, allergic reaction, pneumonia, hypoxia (low oxygen level), injury to the teeth, irregular heart rhythms, spasm of the esophagus or larynx, and death (< 1/10,000).

[X] N/A Non-anesthesiologist-Delivered Moderate Sedation: I understand that I will receive sedation through my intravenous (IV) line in order to help me feel more comfortable during my procedure. This sedation is not general anesthesia and is not administered by an anesthesiologist. With this sedation, I may still be aware of what is happening. There are risks to sedation, including (but not limited to) allergic reactions, drug reactions, bleeding, blood clots, breathing problems that require a breathing tube, nerve injury, brain damage, infection, or loss of bodily function or life

[   ] I refuse to let the hospital give information to the manufacturer and/or FDA.

Trainees & Observers: Beth Israel Deaconess Medical Center is a teaching facility. This means that healthcare trainees such as resident physicians and students may be involved in or observe my care. All trainees are supervised by professional staff.

Patient Consent: My questions have been answered. I have read and understood the content of this form. I consent to treatment and medical care.

X _____ or X _____

Patient (or person authorized to sign for patient) and relationship to patient, and date.

I have explained the above statements to the patient and answered all questions.

_____ MD _____ MD

Signature   Print name

TRANSESOPHAGEAL PRELIMINARY REPORT FORM

12/10/09 v11

BETH ISRAEL DEACONESS MEDICAL CENTER

Boston, Massachusetts 02215

TEE PRELIMINARY REPORT FORM

Date: ___ / ___ / 20___

Indication(s): AF/LA throm SOE Endocarditis Dissection Other: _____

Operators:

Sedation: Versed _____ mg Fentanyl _____ mcg   Other: _____

Antisialogogue: _____ 0.1 mg _____ 0.2 mg glycopyrrolate IV

Anesthesia: Viscous lidocaine 10% lidocaine spray

Complications: None _____

Findings: No SEC or thrombus in LA/LAA/RA/RAA _____ LAA ejection velocity

Interatrial septum _____ to 2D and color Doppler

_____ mitral valve _____ veg/abscess _____ mitral regurgitation

_____ aortic valve _____ veg/abscess _____ aortic regurgitation

_____ global LV systolic function

_____ Pericardial effusion

_____ aortic plaque (in the _____) to _____ cm

from the incisors

The patient tolerated the procedure well without evidence of complications.

NPO until gag returns. Review/final report to follow. Please call for questions/problems.

_____, MD / #_____

Attending Pager #

INDEX

Note: Italicized page locators indicate a figure/photo; tables are noted with a *t*.